To my parents who brought me into this world.

To my mom, whose loving womb was my first home.

To my daughters, Farheen and Ambreen, who gave me the honor of becoming their mother.

And to all the moms who allowed me to support them during their labor, childbirth, and after, trusted me to take care of their babies, and allowed me to love their babies like crazy.

Preface

"Womb in Bloom" is a labor of love. As a childbirth educator, I focus mostly on Labor, Delivery, Newborn care, and Breastfeeding. I also wanted to walk with the soon-to-be moms and dads on their journey, from when they got pregnant to the end of the trimester.

What a magical moment it is to see those two lines on the test showing a positive result for pregnancy!

There are many ways to celebrate an expectant mom's pregnancy, whether you want to share it with someone special in your life or keep it a secret. I understand that the news is shocking for some as they might struggle to support a baby. Maybe you are a teenager who got pregnant, or you are someone of little means and wonder how you would support a child financially. Maybe you are a mom who is mature in years and is worried about any complications arising during the birth, or maybe you have some health condition that makes your case a high risk.

Take a deep breath in and now slowly exhale. Remember, hundreds of people in this world were in your situation. Their stories are everywhere. Moms have been giving birth to babies for eons. If they can do it, so can you. Ask someone who is the eighth child in their family how young their mother was when she delivered her first child. And how old was she when she gave birth to the 8th child? Yeah, baby, we are made of tough stuff. You've got it! And there is help. You just have to reach out, and it is there. One of the things you need to learn is to ask for help when you need it.

The Womb in Bloom — Your Week-by-Week Pregnancy Companion will help you know what stage of development your baby is in and what you can expect during each week of your pregnancy. You might be taken aback at first by the tiny shrimp-like appearance of the early fetus, but trust me, it is 100% human in the making.

The book includes a short account of each week and points summarizing that particular week. Learn the week-by-week developments of the fetus, the weight, the size, and the length, and any tests you'll need to undergo. Know that not every test is mandatory. Be prepared with some knowledge of what you need, and which test may be optional and could be skipped.

Being pregnant is fun. It's wonderful knowing that the baby growing inside you is the size of a pea or a coin, and then before you know it, the baby is the size of a cantaloupe or a cabbage. And this pregnancy companion gives you a peek into that. The best part of pregnancy for me was when I felt the baby move and kick in my belly (I have two daughters, by the way).

Mystics have discovered that the state of mind the pregnant mother is in during this time is comparable to the state of being in meditation. That is because your attention is focused most of the time "within yourself" on your baby, naturally leading you to be more focused, thoughtful, and mindful. So, enjoy this deep connection to another human being who will soon be in this world and will soon be kicking those tiny legs, crawling, walking, and then running. Sometimes being a frustrating teen and sometimes a sweet angel. May you have a blessed birth! Enjoy the whole journey.

Remember, no matter how tiny the baby is, it is a big soul entering this world. And you are the bridge that the soul passes through. And remember, the baby is always able to sense your emotions. It's impossible to always be in a peaceful and happy state of mind. It is only natural to have feelings of frustration, anger, anxiety, and so forth. However, it is important that you keep bringing yourself towards a more peaceful, less stressed state and seek out help if you need it.

I wish you all the best for an awesome journey toward the birth of your baby. Or babies if you have multiples.

Acknowledgment

Thanks to my daughter Ambreen, who has supported me emotionally and by giving me valuable insights into 'the fonts and colors' I chose for the weekly videos.

I am grateful for the support of my mom, two sisters, and nieces and nephew in all my ventures.

Thanks to my dad, who must be smiling down from heaven on me.

I thank Firdaus Ahmed, my editor, designer, and digital marketer, for lending me her expertise in editing and designing this book.

Special thanks to my sister Hina for all the 'by word of mouth' students she brought me. Couldn't have done it without you, Channa.

Thanks to all the moms who took my course and left wonderful testimonials on my site and to the moms I supported during their childbirth journeys.

Thanks to my friend Victor "Bassam" Demko, who first got me started on this journey of building an "All-in-one online prenatal course" covering "Pregnancy, Labor, Delivery, Newborn Care, and Breastfeeding." I am grateful for Bassam's valuable prep, sales, and marketing advice.

Thanks to Dr. Salikah Iqbal (OB/GYN), who allowed me to observe her in the labor and delivery rooms. Thanks to Effie Pallotta, Prenatal Educator, who let me audit her prenatal classes to learn how to teach moms and dads. Thanks to my Perinatal Support Worker program teachers, Virginia Collins and Debbie Fazio, for training me to become a childbirth educator.

First Trimester

The first trimester starts on the first day of your last period and lasts until the end of week 12.

Weeks 1 and 2

It may seem odd, but a woman is actually not pregnant the first week or two of the time allotted to the pregnancy. Conception typically occurs about 14 days after your last menstrual period begins. To calculate the due date, the health care provider will count forward 40 weeks from the start of your last period.

Having a health checkup with your healthcare provider before deciding to conceive is a good idea. Your ovaries are getting ready to release the egg for possible fertilization by the sperm.

If you're planning to get pregnant this year, now is the time to learn how to prepare for a healthy and happy pregnancy. Don't worry, you have 40 weeks.

You could start taking a prenatal vitamin now or even three months before conception. Even a generic, over-the-counter prenatal vitamin would work just fine. There are many great options out there to choose from. Remember, prenatal vitamins are only a part of a nutritious diet. Maintaining a balanced and healthy diet is of utmost importance during pregnancy.

The truth is, you may be a little nervous about becoming a mother, but it's really not as scary as it seems. In fact, this is a magical time for you and your baby.

What you can expect:

1. Not Pregnant yet.
2. Conception occurs 14 days after your last menstrual period.
3. Get a health check done by your doctor.
4. Ovaries getting ready for possible fertilization.
5. Prenatal vitamins now or even three weeks before conception.
6. Prenatal vitamins are only supplements.
7. Maintaining a balanced and healthy diet is important.

8.   It's normal to feel scared.

9.   Remember, it's going to be a magical time!

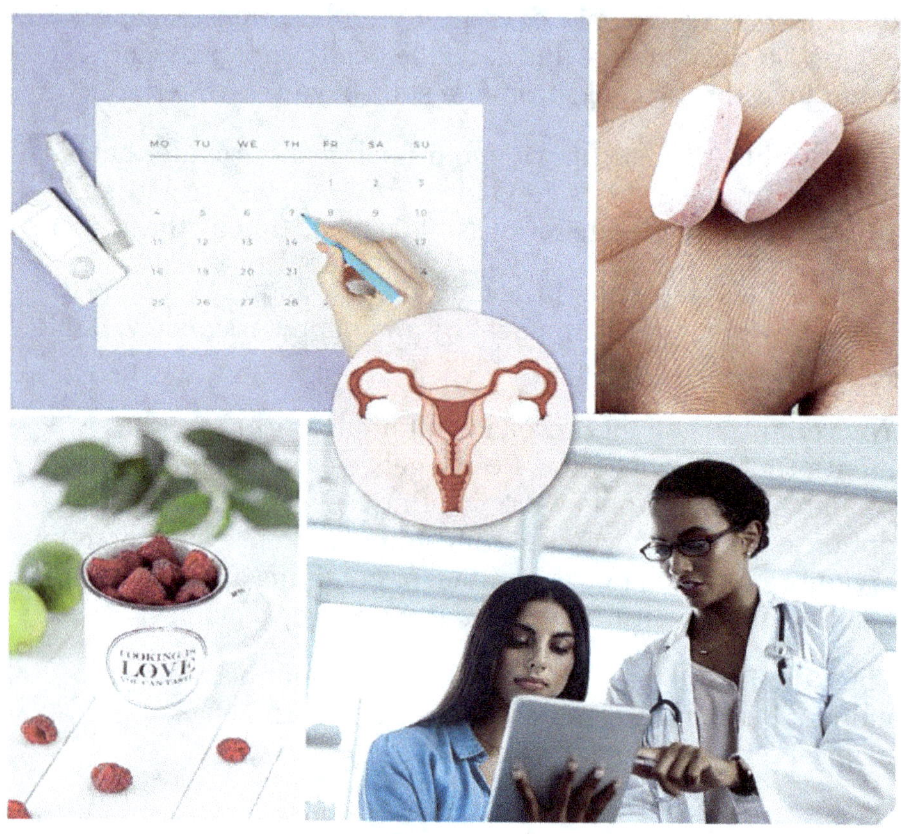

Image Credits: Calendar - Artem Podrez (Pexels), Vitamins - Karolina Grabowska (Pexels), Young woman with Doctor - YuriArcursPeopleimages (Envato), Raspberries - Alexander Mils (Unsplash), Reproductive System Vector - Freepik

Week 3

Fetal development begins soon after conception or fertilization. Following the union of the egg and the sperm in one of the Fallopian tubes, a one-celled entity called a Zygote is formed. If more than one egg is released and fertilized, or if your fertilized egg splits into two, you might have multiple zygotes (twins).

Most zygotes only contain 46 chromosomes, 23 from the mother and 23 from the father. These chromosomes help determine the baby's sex and physical traits. In humans, sex is determined by the combination of X and Y chromosomes inherited from the mother and father.

The zygote travels through the Fallopian tube into the uterus, where it will divide, forming a cluster of cells called a morula, which looks like a tiny raspberry.

You may be slightly nervous about the changes, but you can handle it all. This is a time when you can make a difference in the life of the person you are carrying. It's important to remember that this is a unique time. Don't compare yourself to other mothers or even other new parents. It is just not fair. Remember, your baby absorbs all your emotions.

What you can expect:

1. Fertilization = Conception
2. Union of the egg and the sperm in the Fallopian tube.
3. A zygote is formed.
4. Multiple zygotes (twins, triplets, etc.)
5. 46 chromosomes, 23 from the mother and 23 from the father.
6. Chromosomes determine the baby's sex and physical characteristics.
7. Zygote → Fallopian tube → Uterus
8. Divides and forms cluster of cells - Morula.

9.   Looks like a raspberry.
10. Remember, you can do it!

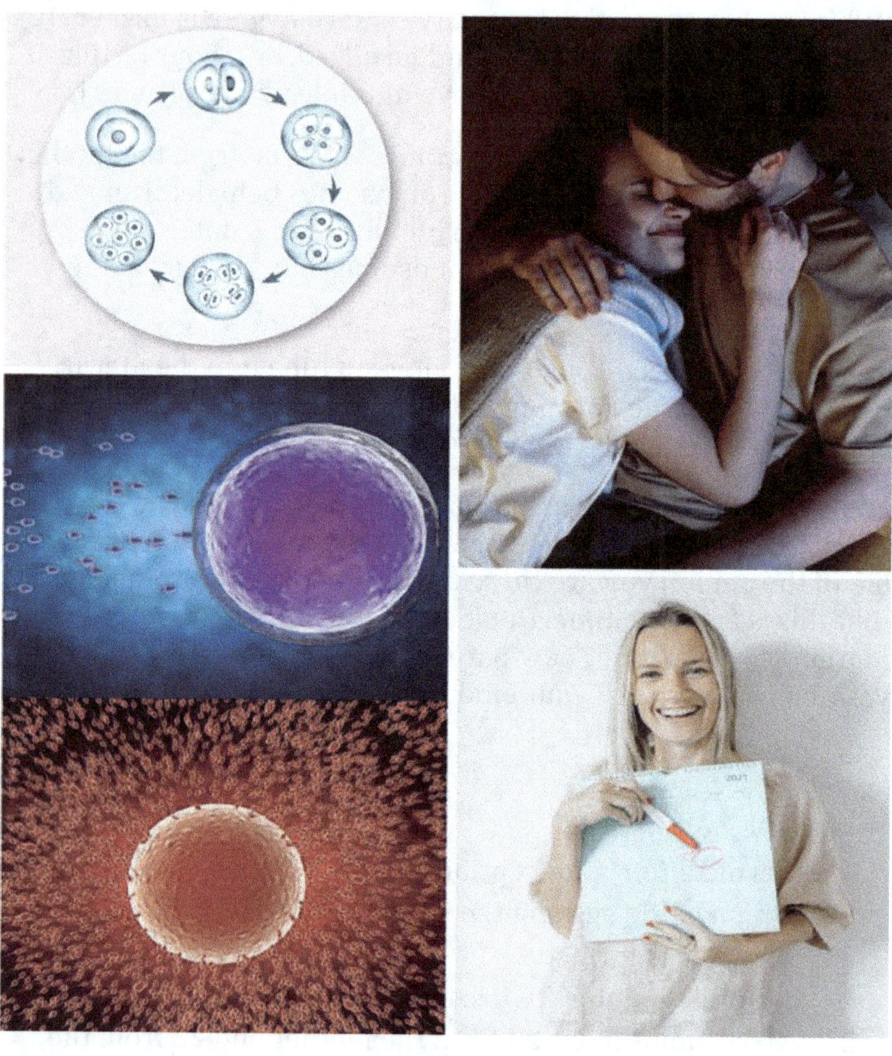

Image Credits: Embryo Cell Division Cycle - Marina (Adobe Stock Photos), Happy Couple - cottonbro (Pexels), Sperm with Ovum (Blue and Red) - phonlamaiphoto (Adobe Stock Photos), Woman with a calendar - nataliya-vaitkevich (Pexels)

Weeks 3 and 4

The cell division that creates a fertilized egg (embryo) is called cleavage. When the cell divides, it divides not only its cytoplasm but also the DNA of that cell. The rapidly dividing ball of cells — known as a blastocyst — has begun burrowing into the uterine lining (endometrium). This process is called implantation. The first stage of implantation is called attachment. Once the blastocyst is close to the endometrium, it begins to push into the uterine lining. Once inside, the blastocyst forms an attachment to the endometrial lining of the uterus.

Within the blastocyst, the inner group of cells will become the embryo. The outer layer will give rise to part of the placenta, providing nourishment throughout the pregnancy.

By the end of this week, a home pregnancy test will usually be able to tell you whether you are pregnant. Congratulations!

Be sure to contact your healthcare provider to determine when you should see him or her for your first prenatal appointment. This generally happens between 8 to 10 weeks after your last menstrual period. Ask your doctor when to schedule an ultrasound for your first visit.

What you can expect:

1. Cleavage of Fertilized Egg.
2. Implantation = Blastocyst. Burrows into the uterine lining.
3. Attachment.
4. Blastocyst → Embryo
5. Outer layer → Placenta
6. Placenta provides nutrition to the baby.
7. Pregnancy test.
8. You are pregnant! Congratulations!
9. Contact your doctor.

10. Size - Poppy Seed

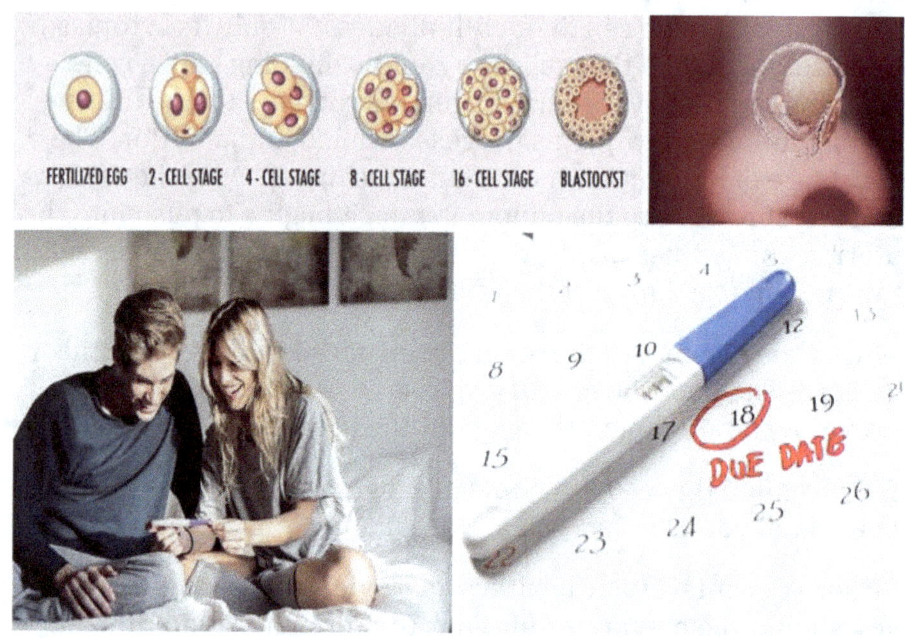

Image Credits: Cell Division Cycle - brgfx (freepik), Red Embryonic Picture - Sciepro (Adobe Stock Photos), Couple with Pregnancy Test - davidpradoperucha (Envato), Due Date - wutzkoh (Envato)

Week 5

The levels of human chorionic gonadotropin (HCG) rapidly rise during pregnancy. HCG triggers the release of hormones from the ovaries that tell the body not to menstruate anymore and stimulates the development of the placenta. It also tells the brain that a new life is growing inside the woman.

The embryo is made of three layers. The top layer gives rise to the skin, your baby's central and peripheral nervous systems, eyes, and inner ears. The middle layer of cells will form the foundation for your baby's heart, circulatory system, bones, ligaments, kidneys, and reproductive system. The innermost layer of cells forms the lungs and the intestines.

As cells from the embryo grow into tissues, they will give rise to all the organs of the developing fetus.

Your baby's tiny heart is beginning to beat and pump blood, the organs are beginning to develop, and limbs are beginning to appear as tiny buds.

Now is the best time to consider what type of childbirth education classes you'd like. There are plenty of options for prenatal classes, and the right class can empower and equip you with the right knowledge to help make your birth less painful and a more fulfilling experience.

What you can expect:

1. HCG levels rise.
2. Menstruation stops.
3. Placenta develops.
4. Embryo - 3 layers.
5. 1st layer → skin, nervous system, eyes, and inner ears.
6. 2nd layer → heart, circulatory system, bones, ligaments, kidneys, and reproductive system.
7. 3rd layer → lungs and intestines.

8.   Cells → Tissues → Organs
9.   The heart pumps blood.
10.   Limbs look like tiny buds.
11.   Size - Grain of Rice.

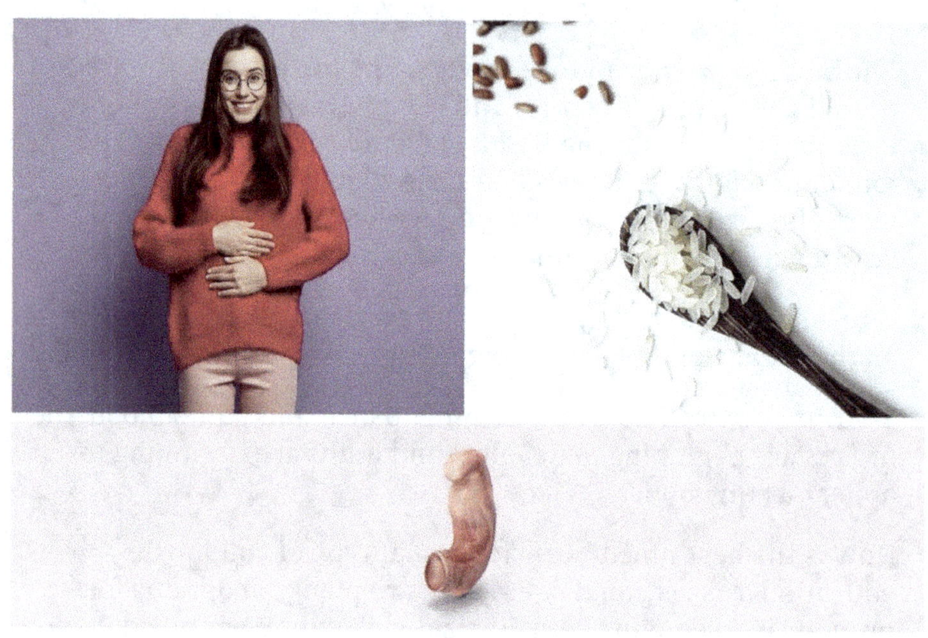

Image Credits: Joyful Woman - Wayhome Studio (Adobe Stock Photos), Rice Grain - Polina Tankilevitch (Pexels), Human Embryo Fetus - PixelSquid360 (Envato)

Week 6

Growth is rapid this week. The neural tube along the back is closing. The nervous system begins developing as the embryo develops. At this point, the main organs, including the brain and spinal cord, are starting to form. The heart and other organs are also starting to form.

The tiny buds that will become the arms are starting to grow. The baby's body is becoming C-shaped as it begins to develop. Now that your baby is about a quarter of an inch (6mm) long, its nose, eyes, mouth, and ears are starting to form.

Now is the best time to consider what type of childbirth education classes you'd like. There are plenty of options for prenatal classes, and the right class can empower and equip you with the right knowledge to help make your birth less painful and a more fulfilling experience. The more prepared you are, the more confident you will be.

What you can expect:

1. Rapid growth.
2. The neural tube closes.
3. The nervous system, brain, spinal cord, heart, and other organs begin to form.
4. Arm buds start to grow.
5. A quarter of an inch.
6. Size of a Sweet Pea.
7. The nose, eyes, ears, and mouth start to form.
8. What type of childbirth or prenatal classes would you like to take?
9. Online, self-paced classes?
10. Or in-person classes?

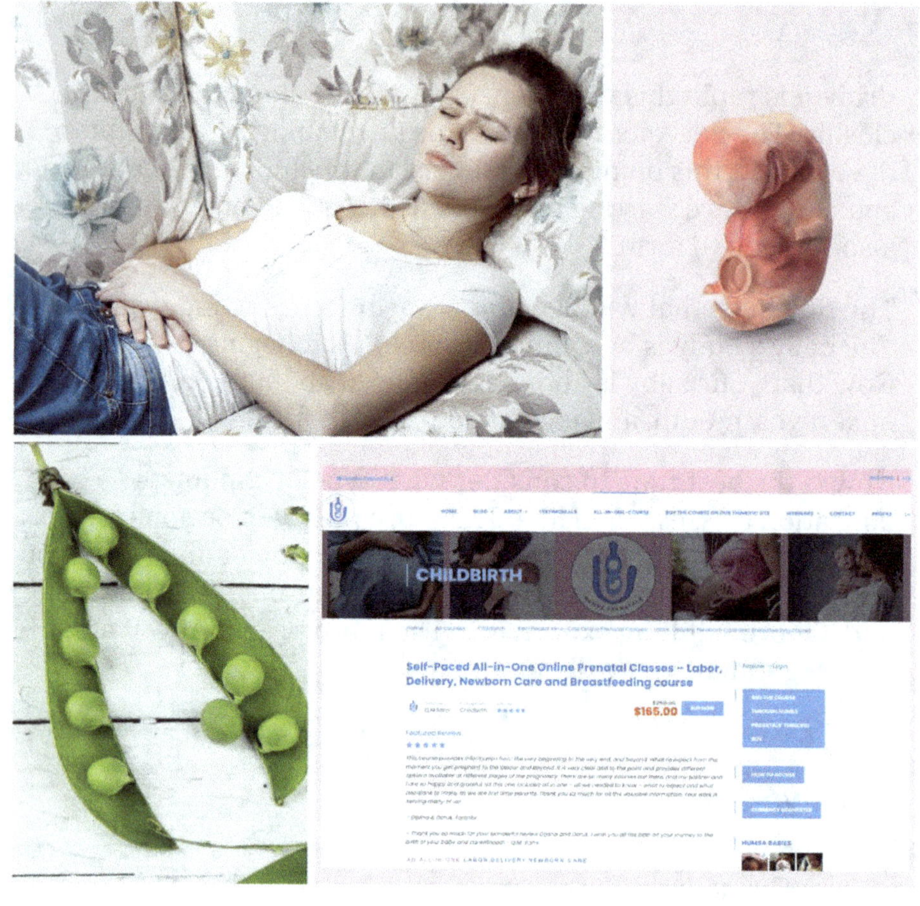

Image Credits: Woman Resting - Khosrork (Adobe Stock Photos), Human Embryo Fetus - PixelSquid360 (Envato), Peas - r-khalil (Pexels), Prenatal Classes Website - humsaprenatals.com

Week 7

As your child grows, their head and brain continue to change in size, and the face starts to take shape. Concave pockets that will grow into nostrils become visible, and the retinas, which later get pushed back into the eyes, start to form.

The embryo's lower limb buds that will eventually turn into the legs begin to emerge, and the arm buds that appeared a week ago begin to take shape. You'll most likely start experiencing some discomforts of pregnancy, like nausea, sensitivity to the smell of different foods, food aversions, frequent urination, and extreme exhaustion.

Try to experiment and see what foods you can keep down without vomiting. This is when your baby's brain and nervous system are developing. It is crucial that you get proper nourishment.

You might get ready for that first prenatal appointment with your doctor. Your childbirth class may be able to point you toward drafting a rough copy of your birth plan. Creating one may help you understand which direction you envision your childbirth. You can begin to craft your birth plan by making a list of your desired outcomes.

Birthing centers and home birth can provide a great option for families that wish to avoid the hospital environment. In contrast, other options like hospitals allow parents access to modern medical services in emergencies where interventions become necessary.

Check out some birthing centers, talk to some midwives, and see what they offer. You can also schedule a tour of the birthing unit at the nearest hospital.

What you can expect:
1. The heart and the brain change in size.

2. The face starts forming.
3. Nostrils and retina start forming.
4. Lower limb buds appear.
5. Arm buds take shape.
6. Nausea, sensitivity to smell, food aversions, frequent urination, and exhaustion.
7. It is crucial to have nourishment in your diet.
8. Start making a birth plan.
9. Where would you like to give birth?
10. Check out a birthing center or hospital and schedule your first prenatal appointment with a doctor.

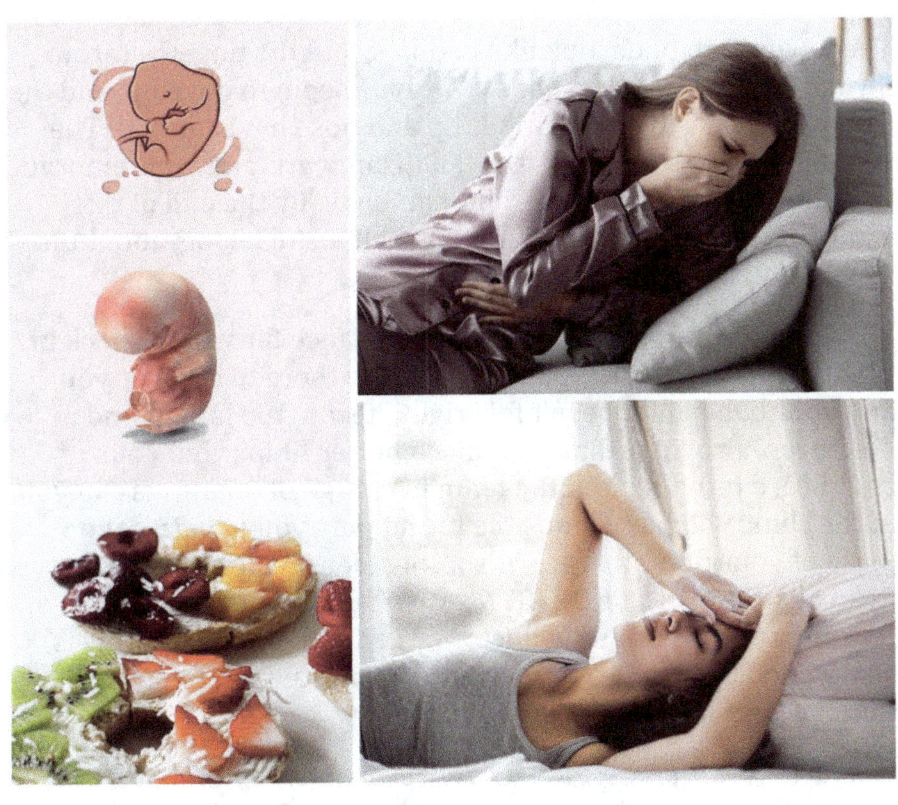

Image Credits: Woman with nausea - Pixel-Shot (Adobe StockPhotos), Embryo - Freepik, Human Embryo Fetus - PixelSquid360 (Envato), Bagel with fruits - Jane Doan (Pexels), Tired woman - Andrea Piacquadio (Pexels)

Week 8

The lower limb buds look like paddles, and the fingers start to form, and the legs take shape. The eyes begin to develop, and the ears become visible. The upper lip and nose have formed. The trunk and neck straighten, the tail disappears, and your embryo will start looking more like a human baby. By the end of this week, the embryo is approximately half an inch long, about the size of a quarter (coin).

Your prenatal appointment is a good chance for you to check in with the doctor and the staff that will be there to care for you and your baby. If it doesn't feel right, it's not too late to find a healthcare provider that feels like a better fit for you. Your healthcare provider and the team in charge of taking care of you at the clinic will be responsible for helping you navigate the maze of your prenatal care. Also, consider if you would like to be in an obstetrician's or OB/GYN's care during your pregnancy, or do you prefer your family doctor or general physician? This is also a good time to discuss any first-trimester screening tests that the doctor recommends.

Fun fact - Not every test the doctor recommends is mandatory, though they are made to sound like they are. Do your research, know your facts and rights, and decide.

What you can expect:

1. Fingers and legs are taking shape.
2. Eyes develop, and ears appear.
3. Upper lip and nose form.
4. Trunk and neck straighten.
5. Tail disappears.
6. Half an inch long.
7. Size - a Quarter Coin.
8. Deciding upon which doctor to see.
9. What first-trimester tests does your doctor recommend?

10.   Are they all necessary?

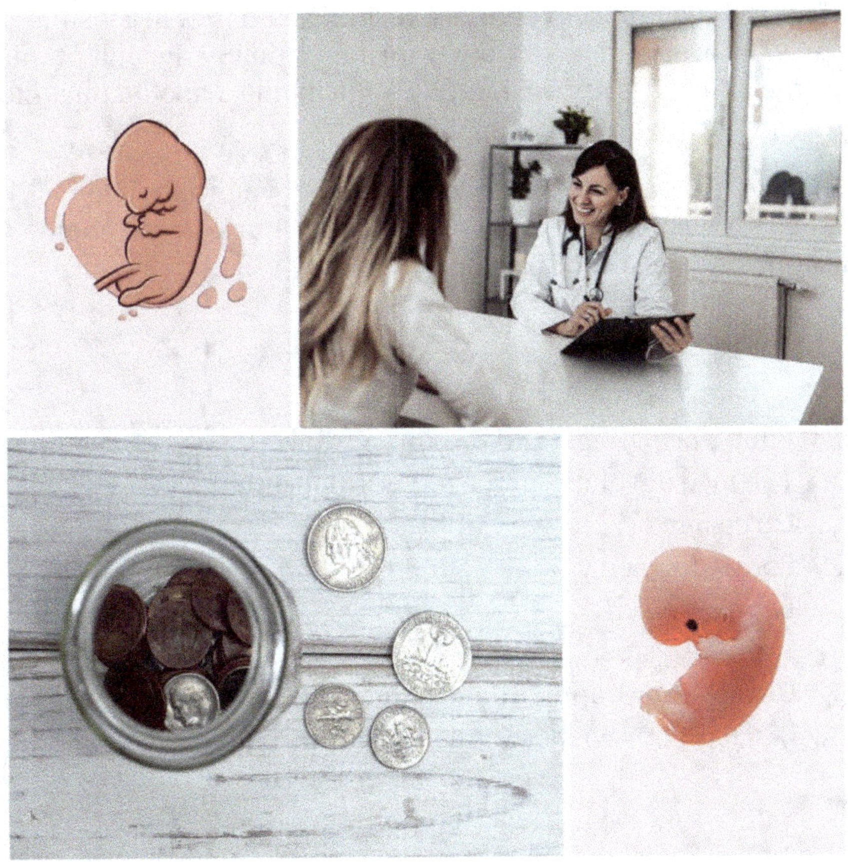

Image Credits: Embryo - Freepik, Woman with Doctor - bnenin (Adobe Stock Photos), Coins - miguel-á-padriñán (Pexels), Reddish Embryo - Sciepro (Adobe Stock Photos)

Week 9

During this week, your baby's arms grow, and elbows are visible. The face is developing, eyelids are forming, and toes are visible. The head is large and has a poorly formed chin. By the end of this week, the embryo is approximately ¾ inch long. Can you imagine that? A miniature human being in the making.

An ultrasound or Doppler device may detect your baby's heartbeat. It's important that you talk with your partner about your hopes, wishes, and plans for your baby's birth.

What you can expect:

1. Baby's arms, legs, and toes are visible.
2. The face develops, and eyelids are forming.
3. Large head.
4. Poorly formed chin.
5. Length ¾ inch.
6. Size of a grape.
7. Ultrasound/Doppler detects heartbeat.
8. Discuss your wishes for childbirth with your partner.

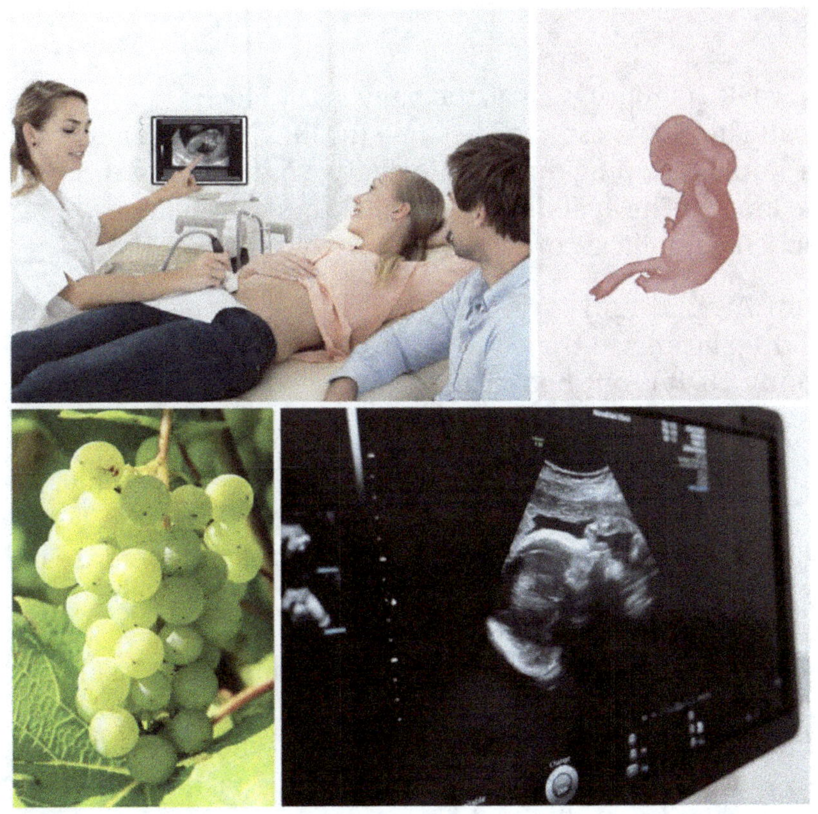

Image Credits: Ultrasound Session - Andre Popov (Adobe Stock Photos), Fetus - humsaprenatals.com, Grapes - Pixabay, Ultrasound Picture - Mart Production (Pexels)

Week 10

During week 10 of pregnancy, the baby's head looks more spherical. The elbows start to become flexible. The toes and fingers stop developing the webbing between the digits and become longer. The eyelids and external ears continue to develop. The umbilical cord is now clearly visible.

Heads up. Around 11-14 weeks, your doctor may suggest a Nuchal translucency ultrasound test to detect Down Syndrome or Trisomy 18. It is optional. The older the woman, the more likely a doctor might suggest this test.

Do your research and discuss it with your partner and family. Be prepared. What does your gut say? Some decide not to go through with the test as they might be more accepting in case the child is born with a developmental disability. It is common knowledge that individuals with Down Syndrome still grow to lead a full and meaningful life despite their condition. Trisomy 18 or Edwards Syndrome is rare. Babies with this condition may be stillborn or might not live long. Still, those who have Mosaic Trisomy may live to adulthood, and those with partial trisomy may live regular lives, albeit with some health problems and developmental difficulties.

The nuchal translucency test is not the most accurate in detecting birth defects. However, the results from the test may lead your doctor to suggest amniocentesis, which is another test done to determine birth defects. Please know that there is always a risk of pregnancy loss with amniocentesis.

What you can expect:
1. The Head is rounder.
2. Elbow movement.
3. Toe and fingers grow longer and lose webbing.
4. Eyelids and external ears develop.
5. Umbilical cord visible.

6.   Size of a strawberry.
7.   Heads up! Your doctor may suggest Nuchal translucency test between 11 - 14 weeks.
8.   It is optional.
9.   Start researching Nuchal translucency ultrasound.
10. Be informed and be prepared to say either yes or no.

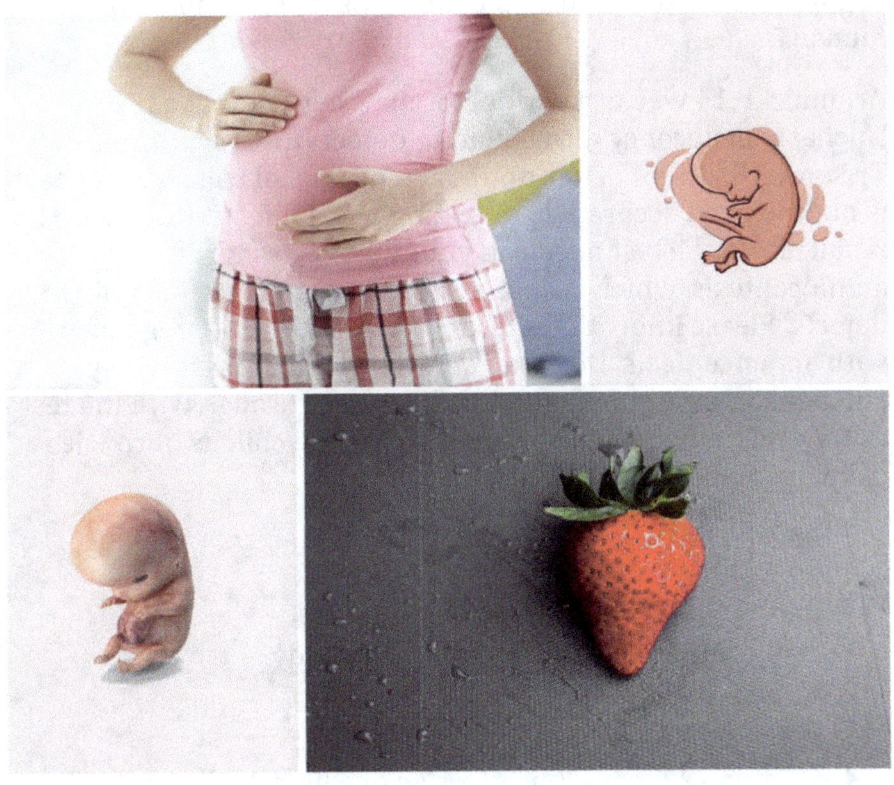

Week 11

During week 11 of pregnancy, the head is still as big as half the body's length. However, the body is about to catch up. At this point, the external genitalia will start developing. Buds for future teeth appear. By now, the fetus is approximately 3 inches long, about the size of a lime, and weighs about an ounce (28g). The hands, feet, fingers, toes, ears, nose, and more features are beginning to take shape, and the baby is looking more and more human.

Around 11-14 weeks, your doctor may suggest that a test, Nuchal translucency ultrasound to detect Down syndrome or Trisomy 18, be done. It is optional. The nuchal translucency test is not the most accurate in detecting birth defects. However, the results from the test may lead your doctor to suggest amniocentesis, which is another test done to determine birth defects. Please know that there is always a risk of pregnancy loss with amniocentesis. Do your research and discuss it with your partner and family. Some decide not to go through with the test as they might be more accepting in case the child is born with a developmental disability.

What you can expect:

1. The head is half the length of the body.
2. Genitalia develop.
3. Teeth buds appear.
4. Fetus - 2 inches long, the size of a lime, 0.25 ounces (7 grams.)
5. Hands, feet, fingers, toes, ears, and nose take shape.
6. Looking more and more human now.
7. Your doctor may suggest Nuchal translucency test between 11 - 14 weeks.
8. It is optional.
9. Do your research.

10. Discuss with your partner and your family.

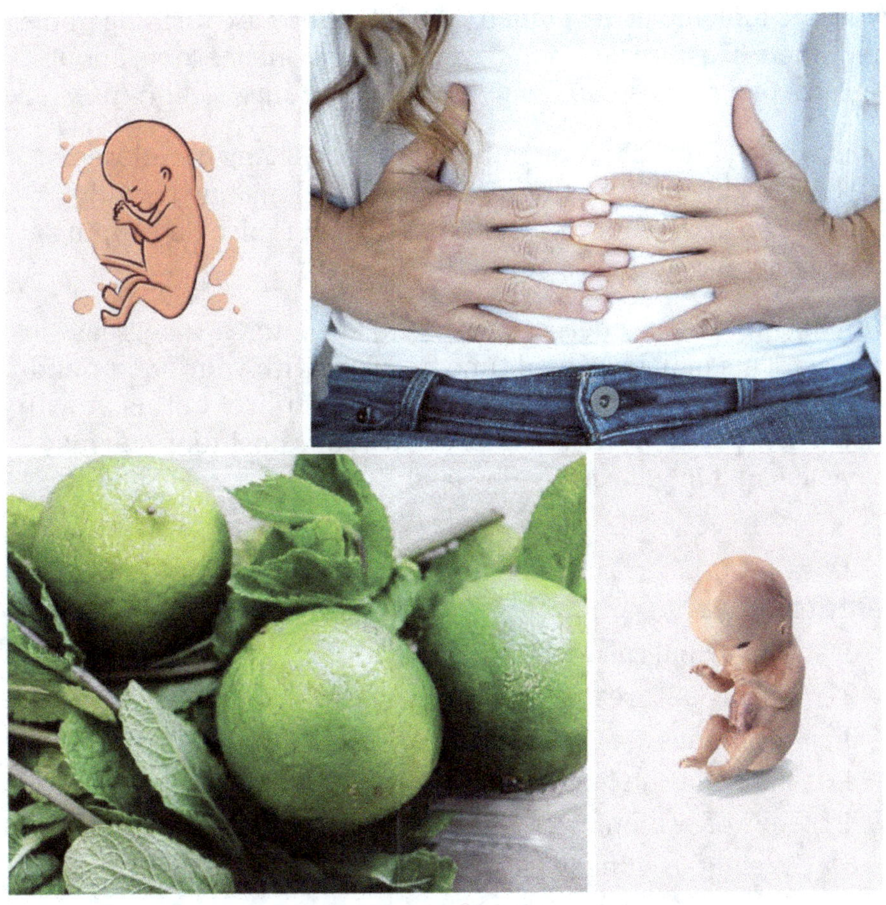

Image Credits: Couple - WavebreakmediaMicro (Adobe Stock Photos), Fetus - freepik, Lime - Lena Kulybaba (Unplash), Human Embryo Fetus - PixelSquid360 (Envato)

Week 12

During week 12, the fingernails are growing, and the facial features look more developed. The intestines are forming in the abdomen. The fetus is about two and a half inches long, about the size of a plum — and weighs about ½ ounce (14 grams).

This week, your baby's beginning to get the hang of reflexes, such as flexing his/her fingers and toes and making sucking motions with the mouth. Your baby's brain is also developing at an extremely rapid pace.

You may feel more energetic now and even notice a decrease in nausea. This may be a good time to check with your doctor and try a prenatal yoga class or establish an exercise routine. It will also allow you to practice some of the labor positions you may have learned in your prenatal class.

What you can expect:

1. Fingernails grow.
2. Facial features are developing.
3. Intestines are forming.
4. 2.5 inches in length.
5. Size of a plum.
6. Weight ½ ounce (14 grams.)
7. Reflexes - flexing fingers and toes.
8. Sucking movements.
9. The brain is developing.
10. The mother has less nausea and more energy.
11. Check out a prenatal yoga class.

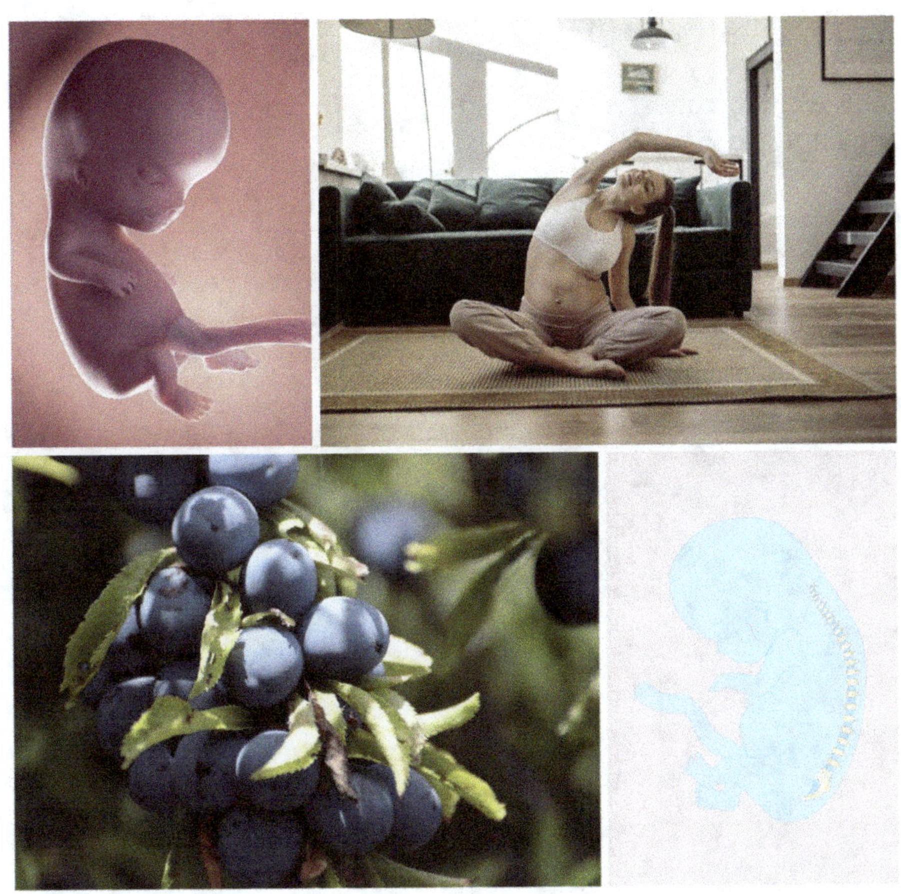

Image Credits: Pregnant Woman doing Yoga - yan-krukov (Pexels), Reddish Fetus - Sciepro (Adobe Stock Photos), Plums - Julian Ackroyd (Unsplash), Infant - Skeleton and bones (Wikimedia Commons - curid=82641170)

Second Trimester

The second trimester is the middle of your pregnancy, from weeks 13 to 27.

Week 13

The fetus makes its urine while developing in the uterus and releases it into the amniotic sac. This week, bones begin to harden, especially in the baby's head, legs, and arms. The skin is thin and transparent. But it will soon thicken.

This might be a good time to consider whether you would like a doula or perinatal support person to assist you during the labor.

If you already had a nuchal translucency test, your healthcare provider may have an Alpha-fetoprotein test done around 16 weeks to screen for neural tube defects. Again, please remember that both these tests are optional. If you did not have the nuchal translucency test, your doctor may recommend a Quad screen test, which is optional. Do your research. The test can only show that there might be a possible birth defect, but it isn't accurate in determining it.

What you can expect:
1. The fetus can produce urine.
2. Released into the amniotic sac.
3. The head, leg, and arm bones harden.
4. Who is on your birth team - Support person?
5. Optional tests - Nuchal translucency, Quad.
6. Alpha-fetoprotein tests coming up in week 16.

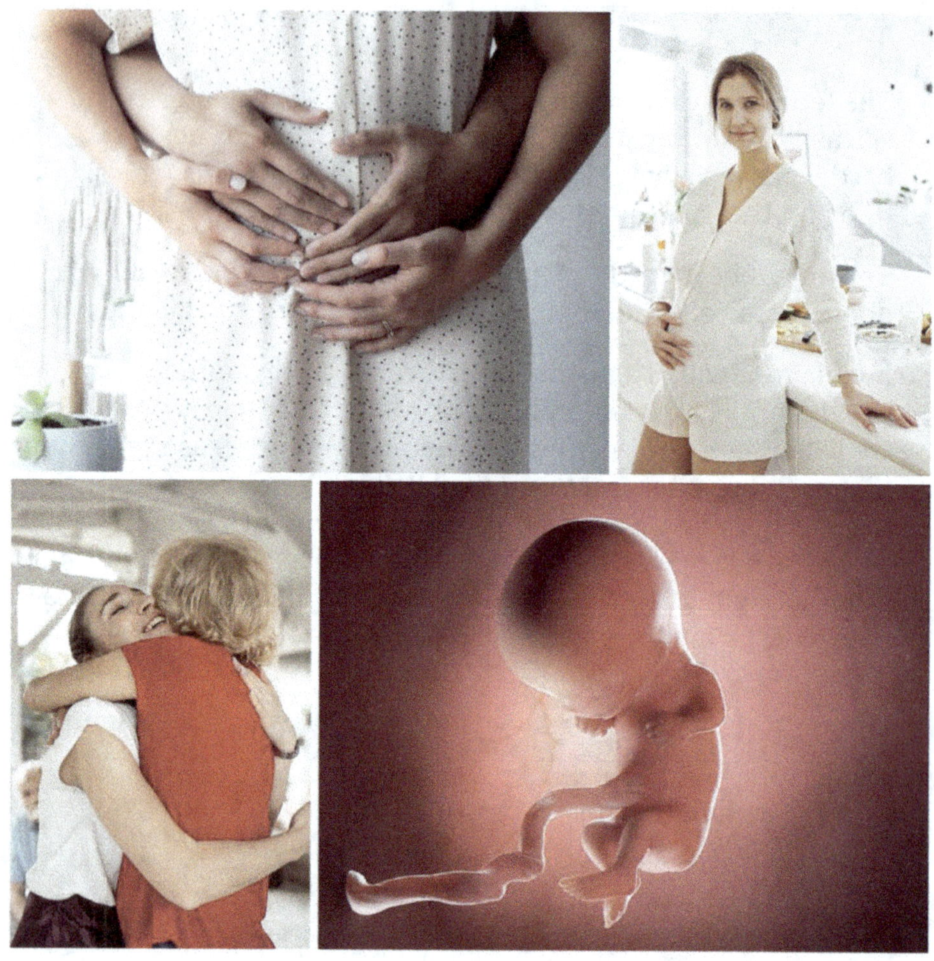

Image Credits: Pregnant Woman being hugged from behind - John Looy (Unsplash), Woman in white - Matilda Wormwood (Pexels), People hugging - Rodnae Productions (Pexels), Redish Fetus Sciepro (Adobe Stock Photos)

Week 14

The fetus's neck is becoming more distinct, and its limbs are well developed. The fetus is approximately 3 ½ inches long — about the size of a lemon — and weighs about 1 ½ ounces (45 grams).

The second trimester is the "honeymoon" stage of pregnancy. Your body is feeling its best during this time, practically glowing. So, enjoy!

In the second trimester, there's less chance of a miscarriage happening than at any other time. You'll see your healthcare provider every four weeks during your second trimester. Consider bringing your partner or labor support person to several appointments to get to know your healthcare provider before your baby's birth.

What you can expect:

1. The neck is becoming more distinct.
2. Limbs well-developed.
3. 3 ½ inches long.
4. The size of a lemon.
5. Weighs about 1 ½ ounces (45 grams).
6. 2nd Trimester: "Honeymoon" stage of pregnancy. Enjoy!
7. Healthcare provider appointment? Every four weeks.
8. Bring your partner along.

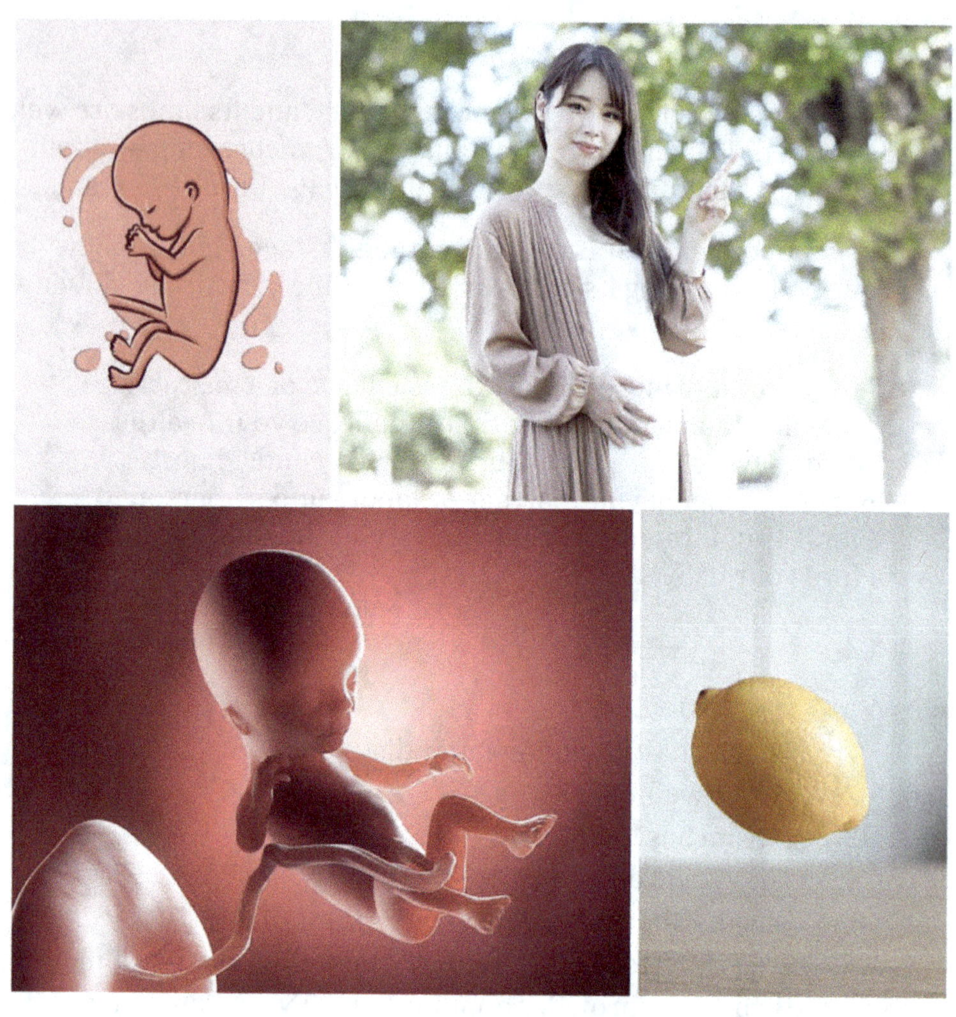

Image Credits: Pregnant woman standing outdoors - buritora (Adobe Stock Photos), Redish Fetus - Sciepro (Adobe Stock Photos), Fetus - Freepik, Lemon - Tara Winstead (Pexels)

Week 15

The fetus is developing very rapidly. Its bone development continues and will be visible on ultrasound images in a few weeks. The hair pattern on the baby's scalp is forming.

You might start to feel Braxton Hicks in the coming weeks. Braxton Hicks is your uterus's way of practicing for the real contractions that will start dilating your cervix during the labor. It's a great time to work on your birth plan with your partner and share it with your healthcare provider.

What you can expect:

1. Rapid development.
2. Bones develop.
3. Hair pattern forms.
4. Possible Braxton Hicks.
5. Braxton Hicks = Practice Contractions
6. Work on your birth plan.
7. Share with your healthcare provider.

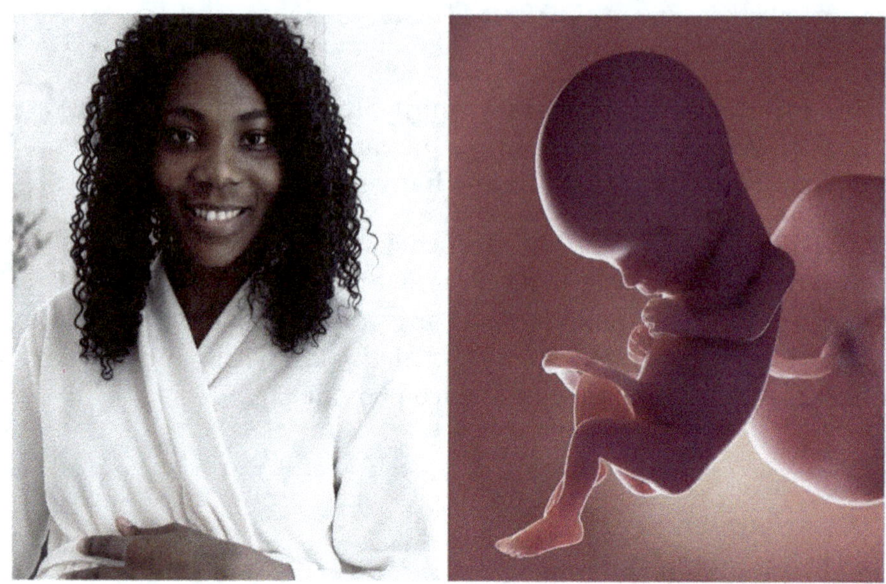

Week 16

The head of the fetus is now upright, and the eyes can slowly move. The ears are nearly in their final position. The limb movements are becoming more coordinated. However, they can be detected during an ultrasound exam but are still too tiny to be felt.

An ultrasound is usually recommended between 18 and 20 weeks to assess your baby's development. Even though you dream about the perfect birth, labor, and delivery can be unpredictable. Read up on cesarean section so that when the time comes to deliver, you will be prepared in case of an emergency.

What you can expect:

1. Head upright.
2. Eyes move slowly.
3. Ears are almost in the final position.
4. Limb movements coordinated.
5. Not yet felt, though.
6. Head up! Ultrasound between 18 - 20 weeks.
7. Read up on C-Section, just in case.

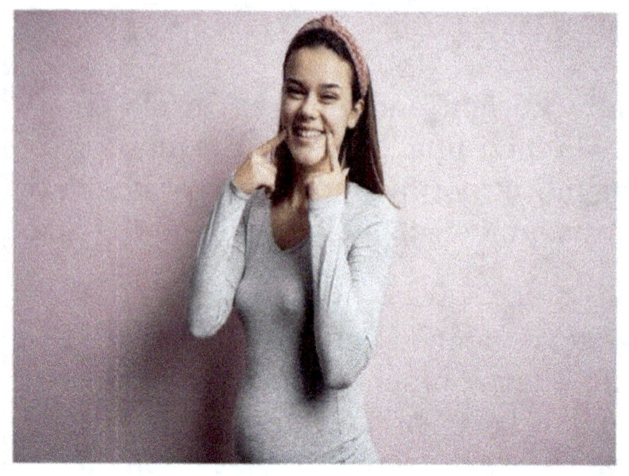 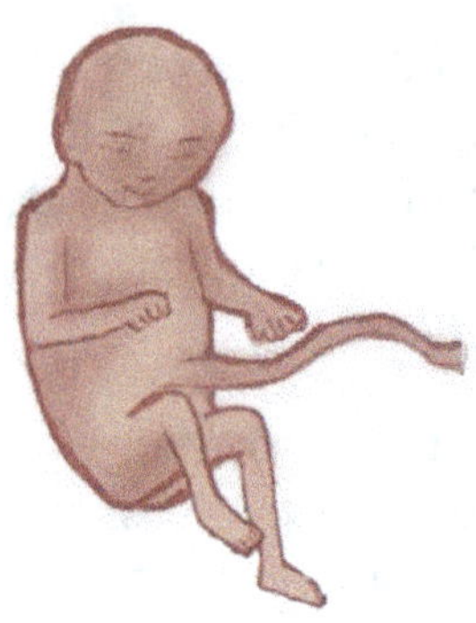

Image Credits: Pregnant woman smiling - Krakenimages (Adobe Stock Photos), Fetus - humsaprenatals.com

Week 17

From now until 22 weeks, you will start to feel the baby move. The fetus in the amniotic sac is becoming more active. It's rolling and flipping.

Toenails begin to grow, and the heart pumps around 100 pints of blood daily.

It might be time to consider what kind of support you need at home after the baby's birth.

What you can expect:

1. You will feel your baby's movement.
2. Active.
3. Rolling, flipping.
4. Toenails grow.
5. Heat pumps - 100 pints of blood daily.
6. Think of what support you need at home after birth.

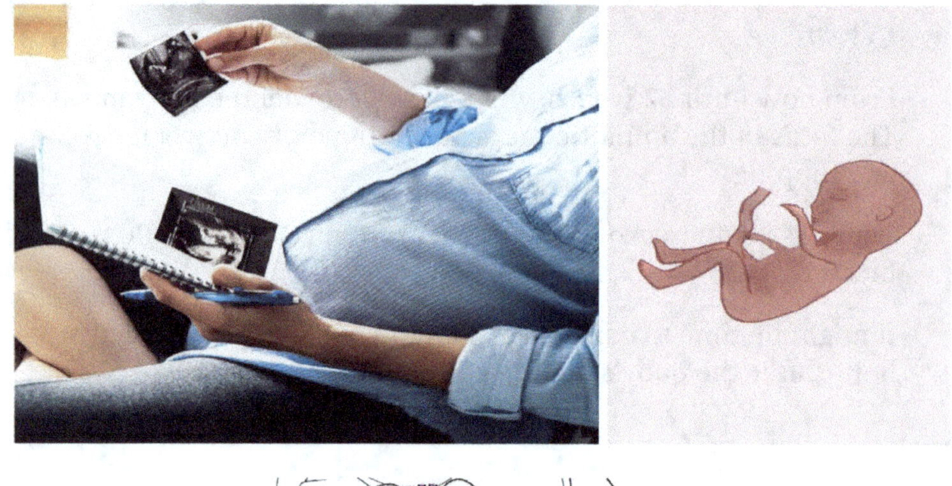

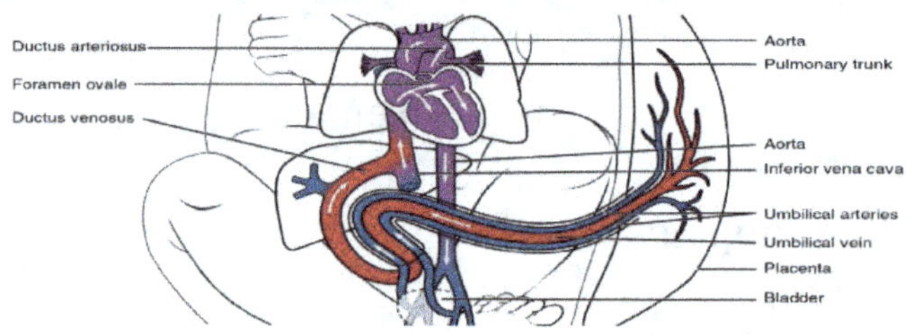

Image Credits: Pregnant woman looking at ultrasound pics - nataliaderiabina (Adobe Stock Photos), Fetus - humsaprenatals.com, Fetus's Circulatory System (Wikimedia Commons - curid=30148296)

Week 18

The ears of the fetus begin to project out on the sides of the head so that the baby might begin to hear. The eyes are developing to face forward. The baby's digestive system begins to work.

Your baby is about 5 ½ inches long and weighs about 5 ounces (142 gm). At this point, your ultrasound technician can tell you whether your baby is a boy or a girl.

What you can expect:

1. The ears are now on both sides of the head.
2. The baby can hear now.
3. The digestive system starts to work.
4. 5 ½ inches long.
5. Weighs about 5 ounces (142 gm).

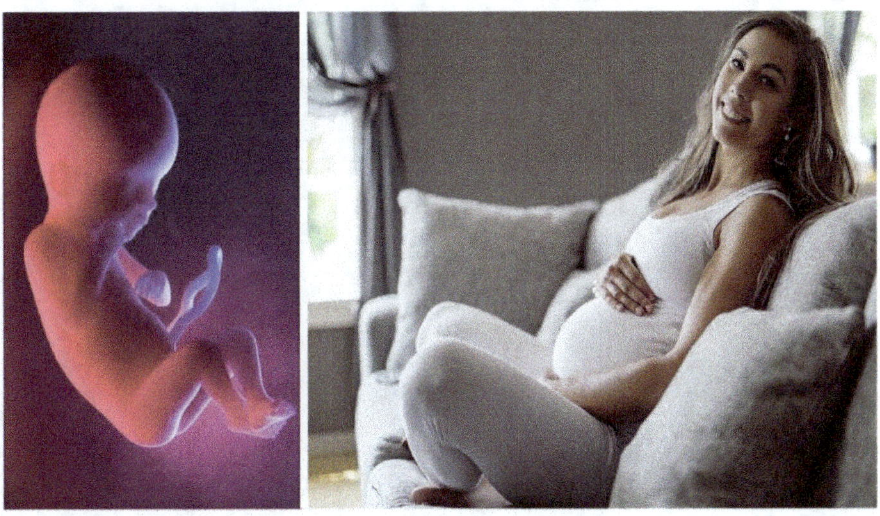

Image Credits: Fetus - Sciepro (Adobe Stock Photos), Pregnant woman sitting on a sofa - Kjekol (Envato)

Week 19

The fetus is covered with a greasy, cheesy coating called Vernix Caseosa.

This coating helps protect the baby's skin from chapping when exposed to amniotic fluid. The growth of the fetus slows down if it is a girl, the uterus and vaginal canal form.

The fetus is approximately 5 ½ inches long — about the size of a mango — and weighs about 7 ounces (200 grams). Your baby may be able to hear your voice by now. You may want to begin taking childbirth classes over the next few weeks.

What you can expect:
1. Vernix = Cheesy coating on the skin.
2. Growth slows down.
3. If it is a female, genitalia develop.
4. 5 ½ inches long.
5. Size of a mango.
6. Weighs about 7 ounces (200 grams).
7. Baby can hear your voice now.
8. Enroll in childbirth classes in the next few weeks.

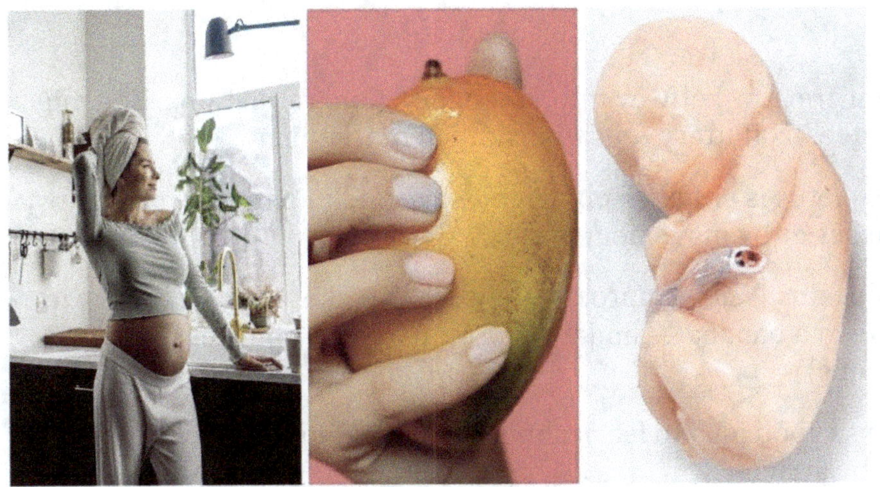

Image Credits: Pregnant woman - yan-krukov (Pexels), Mango - cottonbro (Pexels), Model of Fetus – Sinhyu (Adobe Stock Photos)

Week 20

You are now halfway into pregnancy. Congratulations! You might be feeling fluttery sensations called quickening.

The fetus is either sleeping or awake and might wake up by any noises or by movements.

The fetus is now approximately 6 1/3 inches long — about the size of a banana — and weighs more than 11 ounces (320 grams).

It is a good idea to learn about breastfeeding now before the baby arrives.

What you can expect:
1. Halfway there! Congratulations!
2. Quickening = Fluttery sensations
3. Baby sleeps and wakes up.
4. Sensitive to noises or movements.
5. 6 1/3 inches long.
6. The size of a banana.
7. Weighs more than 11 ounces (320 grams).
8. Learn about breastfeeding.

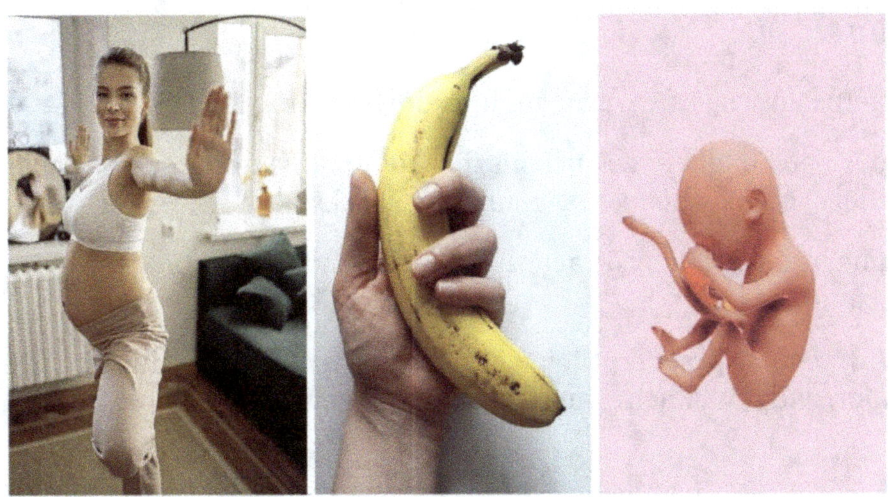

Image Credits: Pregnant woman doing yoga - yan-krukov (Pexels), Banana - kimona (Pexels), Thin Fetus - Peter Schmidt (Pixabay)

Week 21

A fetus now has a covering of fine, downy hair called lanugo.

Your baby might even suck his/her thumb due to the sucking reflex. You may be feeling your baby's kicks now.

Tune into your baby. Practice breathing and relaxation techniques.

With regular practice, they will come naturally to you during labor, and it will help you relax and stay calm.

What you can expect:
1. Downy hair on the skin - Lanugo.
2. Sucking reflex.
3. Sucking the thumb.
4. You may feel kicks.
5. Tune into your baby.
6. Practice breathing and relaxation techniques.
7. Help you stay calm and relaxed.

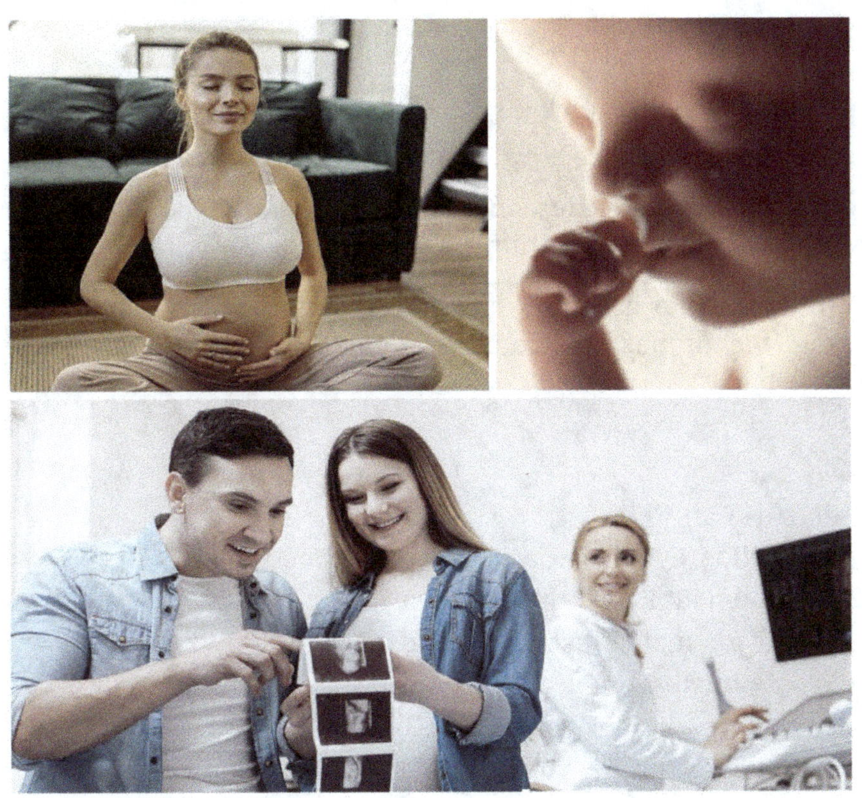

Image Credits: Pregnant woman doing yoga - yan-krukov (Pexels), Fetus - Sciepro (Adobe Stock Photos), Couple - zinkevyich (Adobe Stock Photos)

Week 22

The fetus's eyelids, eyebrows, and hair have now formed. Brown fat, which also generates heat production, is formed.

If it is a boy, the testes descend. Your baby is now 7 ½ inches long and weighs about 12 ounces (0.3 kg).

If your back aches have your partner or support person practice massage techniques. Or stretch your back by leaning over on an exercise ball.

What you can expect:
1. Eyelids, eyebrows, and hair are formed.
2. Brown fat keeps the body warm.
3. If it is a male - testes descend.
4. 7 ½ inches long.
5. Weighs about 12 ounces (0.3 kg).
6. You may have a backache.
7. A partner or support person can practice massage techniques.
8. Practice stretching with an exercise ball.

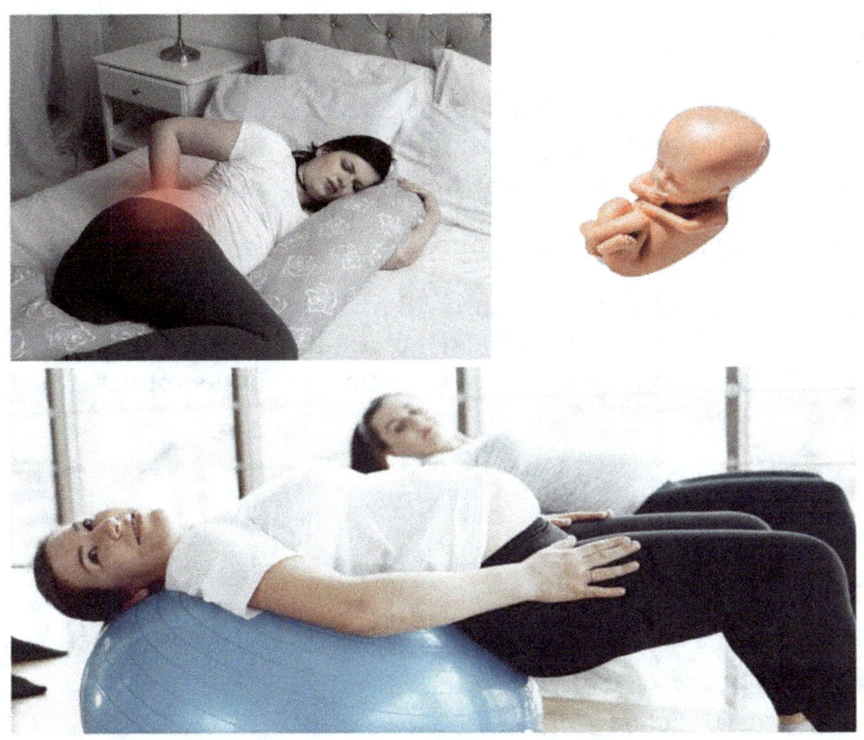

Image Credits: Pregnant woman with back pain - Anna (Adobe Stock Photos), Fetus model - Gina Sanders (Adobe Stock Photos), Pregnant woman lying on exercise ball - gustavo-fring (Pexels)

Week 23

The baby's rapid eye movements begin, and he or she develops creases and ridges in the palms of the hands and soles of the feet. These will later create fingerprints and footprints.

You can feel your baby hiccupping, causing jerky movements.

By now, the fetus is approximately 8 to 10 inches long and weighs about 1 to 3 pounds (0.5 kg to 1.4 kg). Talk about your birth plan and any changes with your partner and support person.

What you can expect:

1. Rapid eye movement.
2. Creases and ridges in palms of hands and soles of feet.
3. Hiccups.
4. 8 to 10 inches long.
5. Weighs about 1 to 3 pounds (0.5 kg to 1.4 kg).
6. Discuss the birth plan with your partner and support person.

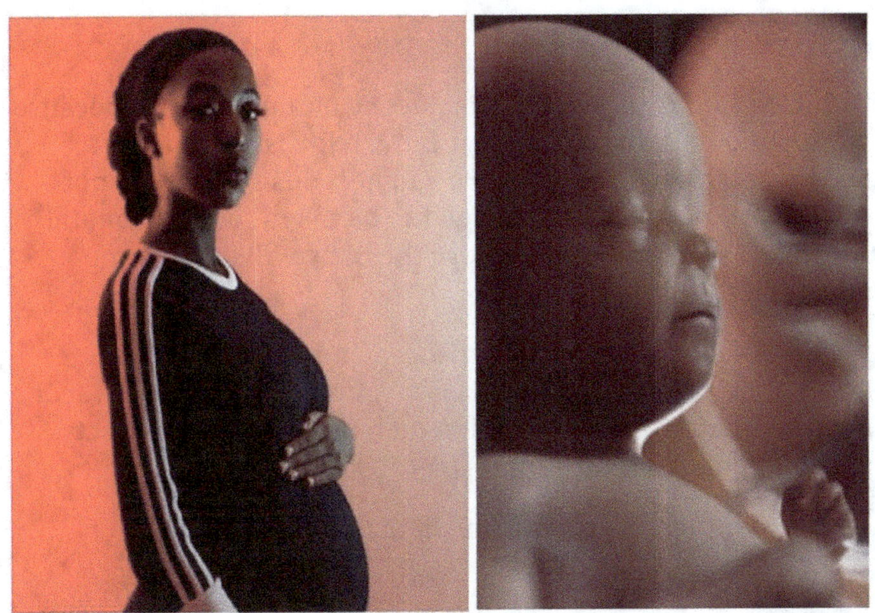

Image Credits: Woman in red background - Toro Tseleng (Unsplash), Fetus with twin in the background - Sciepro (Adobe Stock Photos)

Week 24

The baby's skin is wrinkled, translucent, and pink to red because of visible blood in the capillaries. If the baby is born now, it might survive. Because the lungs and nervous system are not fully developed, the baby will need to be taken to the Neonatal Intensive Care Unit (NICU), where the baby will have proper medical care.

Your healthcare provider may recommend that you have a glucose screen between 24 and 28 weeks to test for gestational diabetes. To learn about gestation diabetes, its causes, effects, and treatment, please visit humsaprenatals.com

You may want to discuss your birth plan now with your healthcare provider.

What you can expect:

1. The skin is wrinkled and translucent.
2. Blood is visible through capillaries giving reddish or pinkish color to the skin.
3. If born is born in week 24, needs NICU.
4. Discuss the birth plan with your doctor.
5. Heads up! Glucose screening - between 24 to 28 weeks.

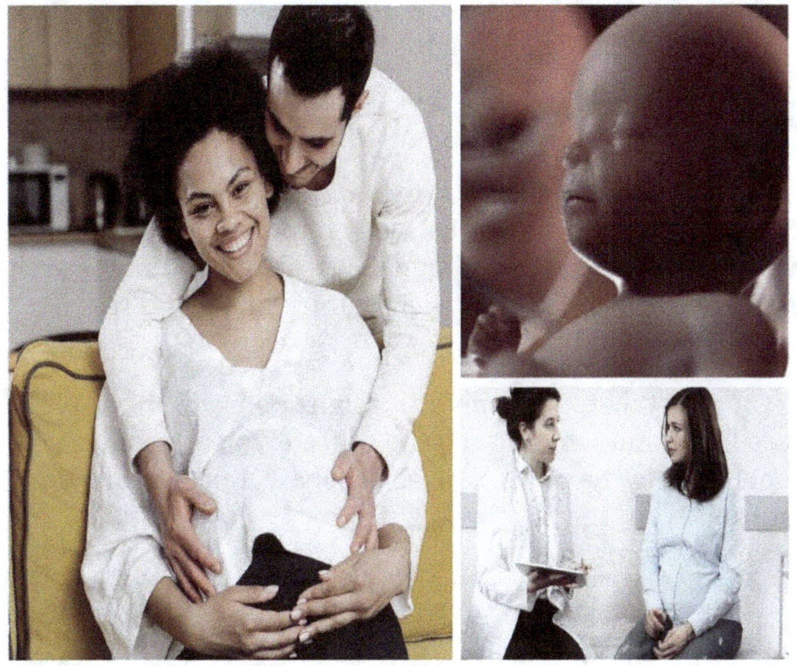

Image Credits: Couple - Ivan Samkov (Pexels), Fetus - Sciepro (Adobe Stock Photos), Woman with Doctor - Mart-Production (Pixabay)

Week 25

Much time is spent sleeping in rapid eye movement (REM) sleep, where the eyes move rapidly, even though the eyelids are closed.

If you are not already, you may be experiencing Braxton Hicks contractions, which is your uterus's way of preparing itself for labor. Your healthcare provider may discuss with you how to tell the difference between Braxton Hicks contractions and real contractions that might be dilating your cervix.

Your doctor may talk to you about the signs and symptoms of premature labor and when to call the office if you are concerned about experiencing them. Also, please check out pre-labor signs and symptoms from the "Labor and Delivery" Masterclass at humsaprenatals.com

What you can expect:
1. The fetus responds to sounds.
2. The fetus kicks and jerks.
3. REM sleep.
4. Continue a nutritious diet.
5. Braxton Hicks = Practice Contractions
6. Uterus preparing for labor.
7. Braxton vs Real Contractions.
8. Ask your doctor about premature labor.

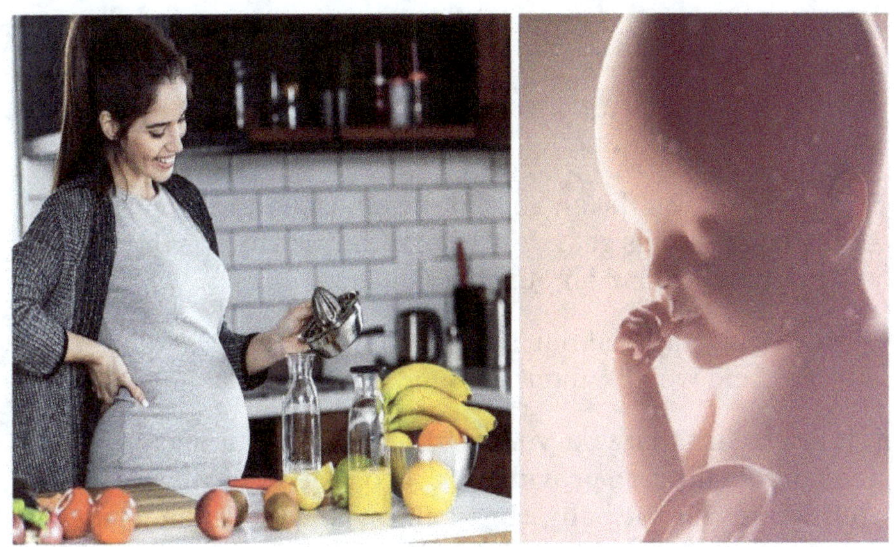

Image Credits: Pregnant woman in the kitchen - lordn (Adobe Stock Photos), Fetus - Sciepro (Adobe Stock Photos)

Week 26

The baby's lungs are growing, and the process of producing surfactant is beginning.

Surfactant allows the air sacs in the lungs to function properly. As the baby's lungs get ready to breathe air after birth, the baby will breathe in small amounts of fluid.

By now, the baby is about 10 inches long, or the size of a cabbage, and weighs about 2 pounds (820 grams).

It is important that you, your partner or labor support person, and your healthcare provider are all on the same page about your wishes for the baby's birth. Know that some knowledge and flexibility, as well as having plans A, B, and C, are the keys to having a satisfactory birth.

What you can expect:
1. Lungs are growing.
2. Surfactant is produced.
3. Surfactant helps air sacs function in the lungs.
4. Preparing to breathe air after birth.
5. Will breathe small amounts of fluid.
6. 10 inches long.
7. The size of a cabbage.
8. Weighs about 2 pounds (820 grams).
9. Important: You, your Partner, your Support Person, and your doctor are on the same page about your wishes.
10. Be flexible. Have a plan A, B, and C.

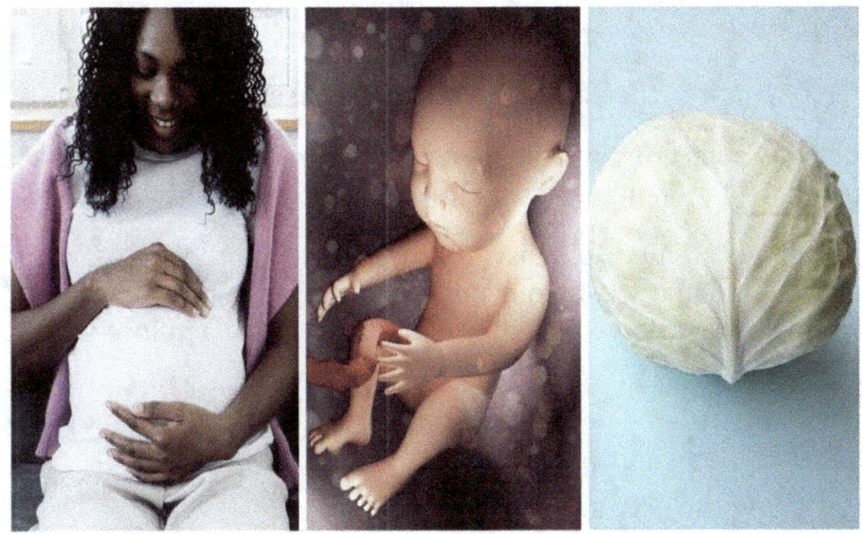

Image Credits: Pregnant woman looking at her belly - Shvets productions (Pexels), Fetus floating - nosorogua (Adobe Stock Photos), Cabbage - laker (Pexels)

Week 27

Week 27 marks the end of the second trimester.

The baby's nervous system is continuing to develop. The fetus is putting on fat; hence, the skin looks smooth and less wrinkly.

The baby is about 3 to 5 lbs. (1.4 to 2.3 kg), and the lungs are beginning to mature. If your initial glucose screening test was high, your healthcare provider may recommend a follow-up test.

What you can expect:
1. End of 2nd trimester.
2. The baby's nervous system continues to develop.
3. The fetus puts on fat.
4. The fetus is less wrinkly.
5. Weighs about 3 to 5 lbs. (1.4 to 2.3 kg).
6. Lungs begin to mature.
7. A follow-up test is recommended if the initial glucose screening test is high.

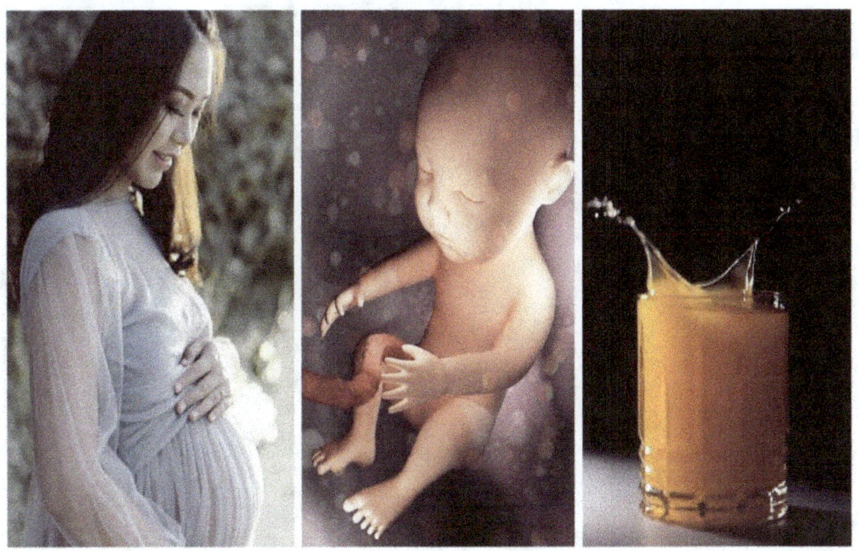

Image Credits: Pregnant woman outdoors - ngakan-eka (Pexels), Fetus floating - nosorogua (Adobe Stock Photos), Orange Juice - Teo-do-rio (Unsplash)

Third Trimester

The third trimester is the last phase of your pregnancy. It begins around week 28 and lasts until you give birth, that is till week 40, but sometimes it goes up to week 42.

Week 28

The baby's eyelids can partially open, and eyelashes have formed. The central nervous system can now direct rhythmic breathing and control body temperature.

Your baby's eyes may be able to see the light that filters through your womb. You'll likely see your doctor every two weeks in the third trimester.

The doctor may recommend getting a RhoGAM injection if your blood type is Rh-.

This will prevent the mom's blood from forming antibodies against the baby's blood in case your baby has an Rh+ blood type. These antibodies can make a baby very sick.

What you can expect:

1. The baby's eyelids are partially open.
2. Eyelashes have started to form.
3. The central nervous system can direct breathing and control body temperature.
4. The eyes can see light filtering through the womb.
5. Doctor - every two weeks.
6. The doctor may recommend a RhoGAM injection if your blood type is Rh-, to prevent the mom's blood from forming antibodies against the baby's blood in case the baby is Rh+. These antibodies can make the baby sick.

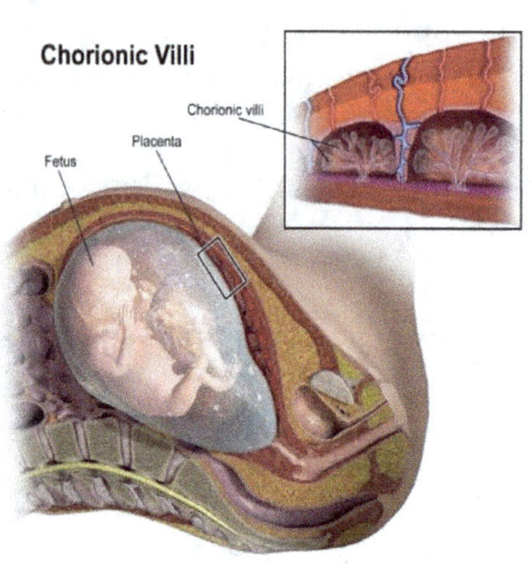

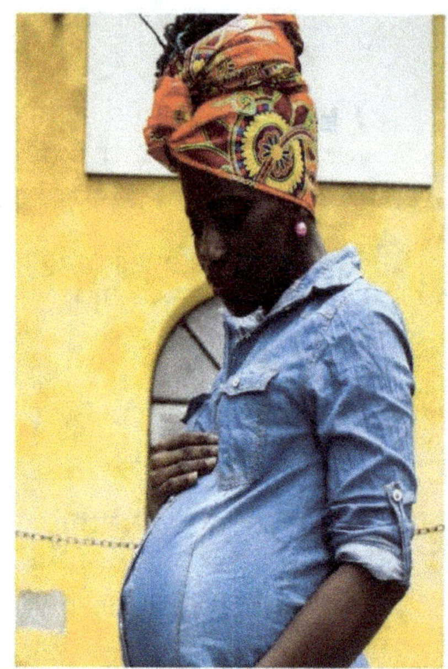

Image Credits: Chorionic villi by Bruce Blaus - (Wikimedia Commons - curid=44897522), Pregnant Woman in blue shirt - Thiago-borges (Pexels)

Week 29

You are now in the home stretch! Your baby can kick, stretch, and make grasping movements.

If you haven't toured the hospital or facility where your baby will be born, now would be a good time to schedule that.

And you can ask for any preregistration forms you can fill out beforehand.

What you can expect:

1. Home stretch!
2. Your baby can kick, stretch, and make grasping movements.
3. Schedule a tour of the hospital or the facility.
4. Preregistration forms can be filled out ahead.

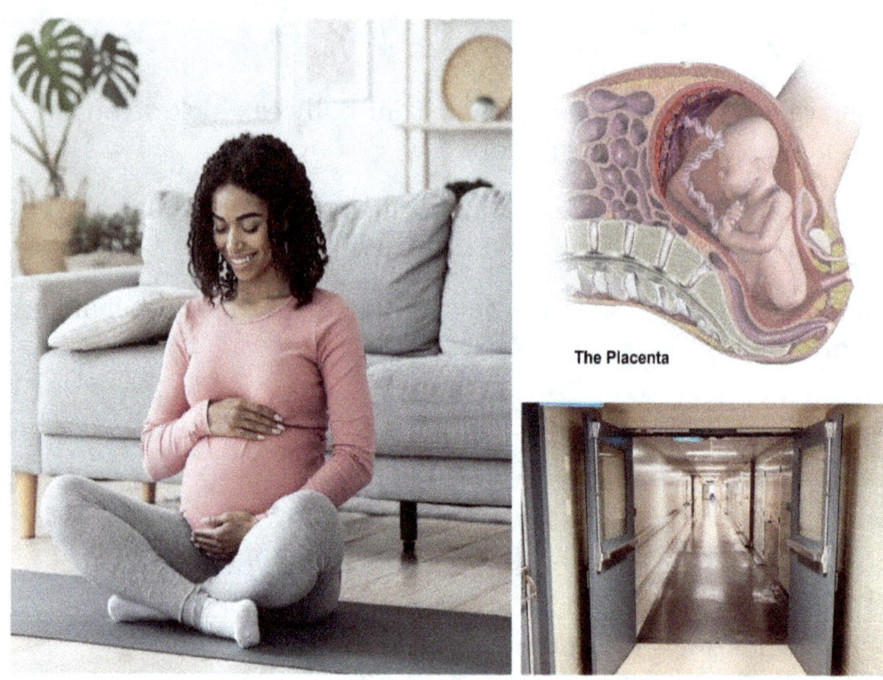

Image Credits: Pregnant Woman - Prostock-studio (Adobe Stock Photos), The placenta by BruceBlaus - (Wikimedia Commons - curid=44897305), Hospital corridor - cory-mogk (Unsplash)

Week 30

By this week, the fetus's eyes can open wide, and he/she may have a good head of hair. Why not use the energy you feel from "nesting instincts" to get some of the things you might want to have during your labor and birth? Buy a birthing ball.

Write that list. Go shopping for that car seat, a stroller, or a crib.

Babies born at 30 weeks may have trouble breathing because the lungs are still not fully developed. The fetus is approximately 10.5 inches long from head to foot and weighs around 3 pounds (1,300 grams).

What you can expect:

1. The baby's eyes can open.
2. May have hair.
3. Mom - "nesting instincts."
4. Make a list.
5. Go shopping - birthing ball, baby bag, diapers, car seat, stroller, or crib.
6. If born at 30 weeks? The baby may have trouble breathing - NICU (Neonatal Intensive Care.)
7. Lungs are still not fully developed.
8. The length is around 10.5 inches.
9. Weighs around 3 pounds (1,300 grams).

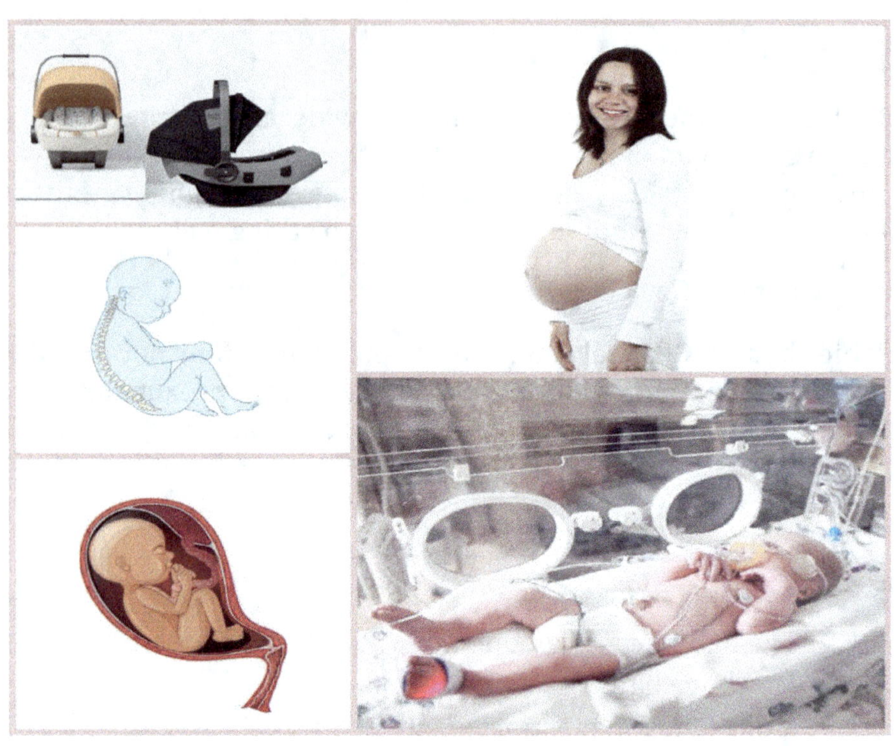

Image Credits: The fetus in the belly - brgfx (Freepix), Baby car seats - Originalmockup (Freepix), Pregnant woman in white (Pixabay), Images related to Fetus newborn baby, Skeleton and bones - (Wikimedia Commons - curid=82641170), Baby in Neonatal care unit - Alexander Grey(Unsplash)

Week 31

The baby may begin to move into the head-down position in preparation for birth unless the baby is a breech.

By now, most of the baby's major development is completed, but still, it needs time to develop some more, and now it's time to put on some weight and strengthen the bones.

You may even feel as if you're gaining weight with every passing day. However, this is a great thing, as it means that your baby continues to develop inside your womb!

If you haven't selected a pediatrician, you could do it now.

What you can expect:
1. Head-down position.
2. In prep for birth (unless breech.)
3. Major development completed.
4. But needs time to develop some more.
5. Time to put on weight and strengthen bones.
6. You may gain weight, but it just means your baby is developing!
7. Time to find a pediatrician.

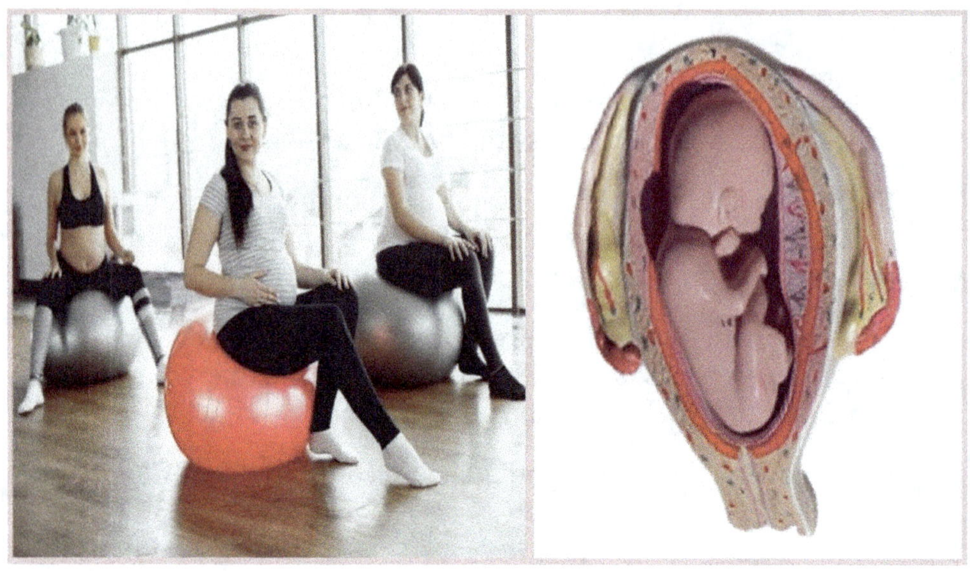

Image Credits: Pregnant women sitting on exercise balls - Gustavo Fring (Pexels), Fetus Model - John Campbell

Week 32

The fetus weighs almost 4 pounds (1.4 kg) and measures about 11-16 inches long. Baby continues to gain weight, and the toenails are visible. The soft, downy hair that has covered the baby's skin for the past few months starts to fall off.

Now would be a great time to review your prenatal class videos or notes to prepare you for the labor.

Just because it feels that the baby has descended and moved downward does not mean the labor will start earlier. Be patient with yourself and the baby. Know that the baby needs time to develop fully.

What you can expect:
1. The fetus weighs almost 4 pounds (1.4 kg.)
2. The length is about 11-16 inches.
3. Continues to gain weight.
4. Toenails are visible.
5. Lanugo begins to fall off.
6. Review your prenatal class videos or notes.
7. Just because the baby has descended does not mean the labor will be early.
8. Be patient with yourself and the baby.
9. Keep in mind that the baby needs time to develop fully.

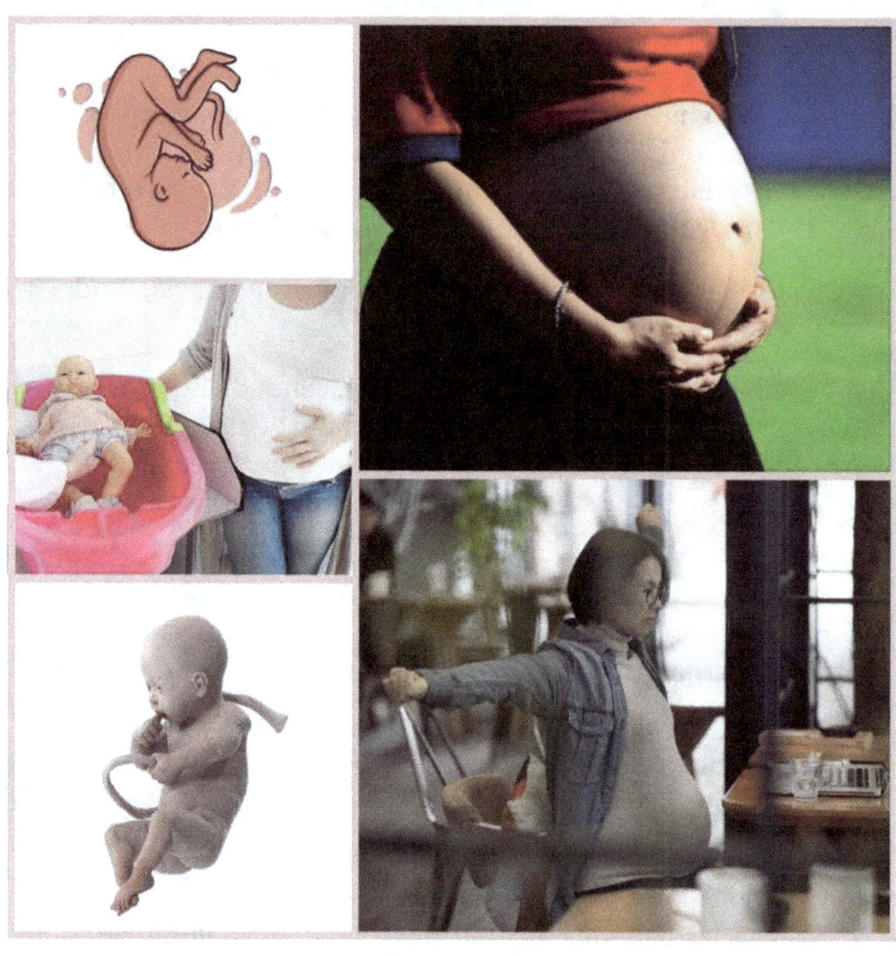

Image Credits: Fetus – Freepik, Pregnant belly - TC.Torres (Pixabay), Prenatal class baby bath - Maria sbytova (Adobe Stock Photos), Human Embryo Fetus - PixelSquid360 (Envato), Tired pregnant woman stretching her arms - Nao (Adobe Stock Photos)

Week 33

The baby's pupils can now change their size and respond to light. The bones are getting stronger, but the skull is still soft and flexible.

You might be feeling a strong urge to work and clean up everything. It's called 'the nesting period.' This surge of adrenaline is nature's way of getting you ready to care for a baby.

Take advantage of the energy by practicing labor positions, breathing, and relaxation exercises.

What you can expect:
1. Baby's pupils change size and respond to light.
2. The bones are getting stronger.
3. The skull is still soft and flexible.
4. Nesting period - the urge to clean and work.
5. A surge of adrenaline - nature's way of getting you ready.
6. Practicing labor positions, breathing, and relaxation exercises.

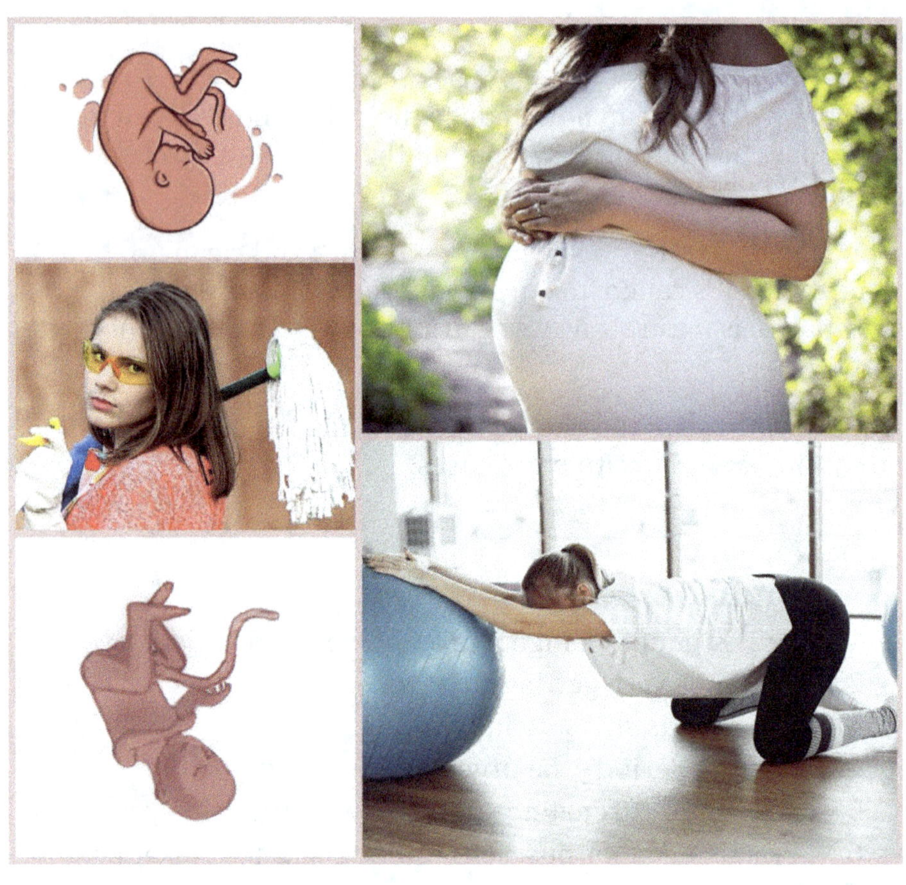

Image Credits: Fetus - Freepik, Pregnant woman in white standing outdoors - ryan-franco (Unsplash), Woman cleaning home - Klimkin (Pixabay), Pregnant woman using exercise ball - Gustavo Fring (Pexels), Fetus - humsaprenatals.com

Week 34

Your baby's fingernails have grown to full size. Your baby is approximately 12 inches long — about the size of a cantaloupe or honeydew melon — and weighs more than 4.5 pounds (2,100 grams).

Though babies born at this age may have fewer long-term medical problems, be patient. Your baby is still building fatty tissue to help regulate the body's temperature after birth. And the nervous system, brain, and lungs are maturing more daily.

This is a crucial time for the baby's growth. You may want to consider taking an infant CPR class now.

What you can expect:
1. Fingernails - full size.
2. The baby is 12 inches long.
3. The size of a cantaloupe or honeydew melon.
4. Weighs more than 4.5 pounds (2,100 grams).
5. Babies born at this age may have fewer long-term medical problems.
6. Still building fatty tissue.
7. Helps regulate the body's temperature after birth.
8. The nervous system, brain, and lungs are still maturing.
9. Crucial time for the baby's growth.
10. Consider taking an infant CPR class.

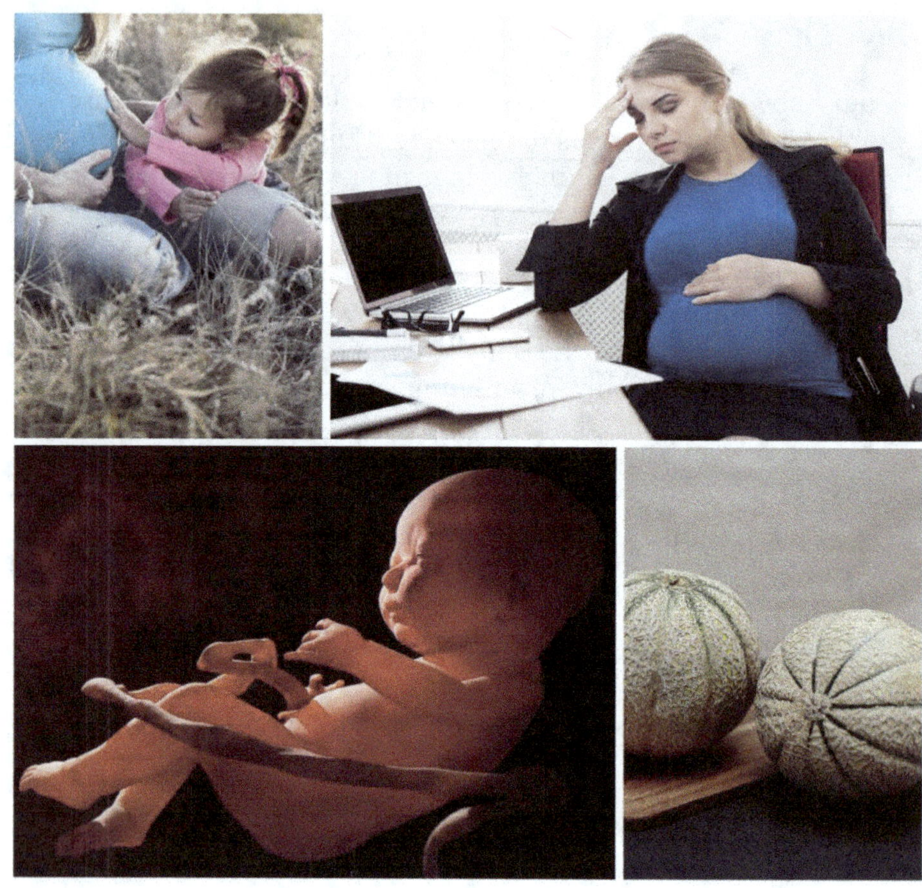

Image Credits: Girl touching mother's belly - anlacreativephotos (Pixabay), Tired Pregnant woman in office - Prostock-Studio (Adobe Stock Photos), Baby floating in the womb - Stock-labden (Adobe Stock Photos), Cantaloupes - cup-of-couple (Pexels)

Week 35

Your baby's skin is becoming smooth and gaining color. The arms and legs are chubbier.

Your healthcare provider might test you for Group B streptococcus bacteria between 35 and 37 weeks, which can infect and make the baby ill if left untreated.

Suppose you test positive for group B strep. In that case, your doctor will suggest starting an early course of antibiotics through IV during labor to protect your baby from infection during the delivery. If that is the case, please talk to your doctor about having a saline lock so that you are not limited to only lying on the bed while laboring.

Movement mustn't be restricted during labor.

What you can expect:

1. Baby's skin is becoming smooth, gaining color.
2. Arms and legs are chubbier.
3. Between 35 and 37 weeks - Group B streptococcus bacteria test.
4. If left untreated, it may infect the baby.
5. Positive for Group B strep? The doctor will suggest an early course of antibiotics through IV during labor.
6. Talk to your doctor about having a Saline lock.
7. Helps not to be limited to only lying on the bed.
8. Important that movement is not restricted during labor.

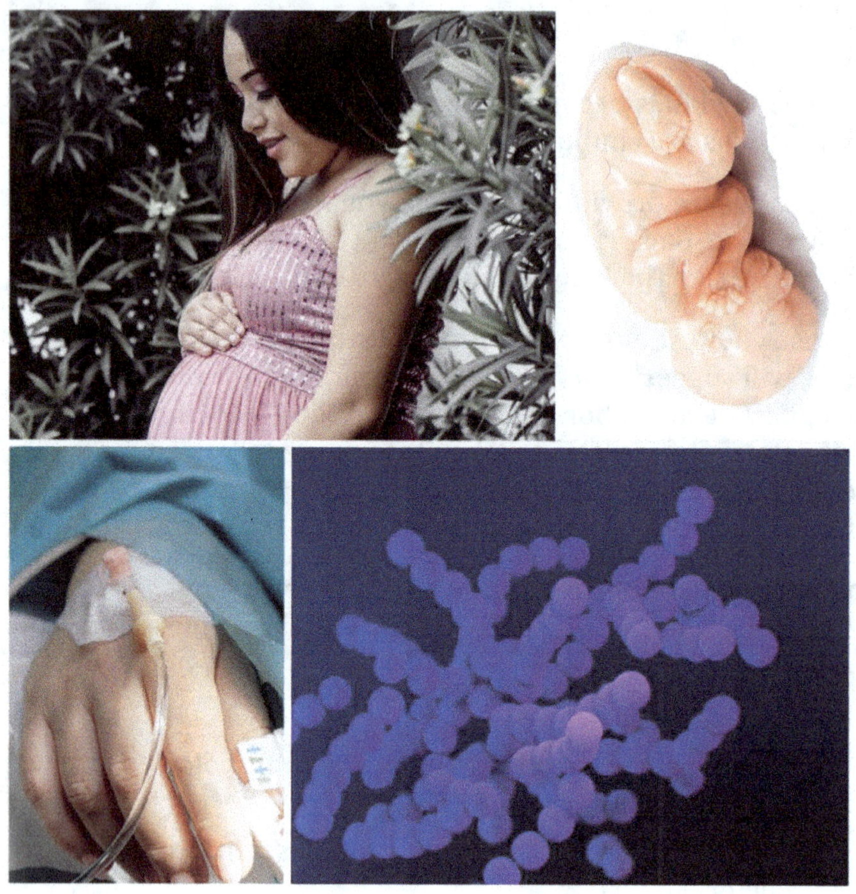

Image Credits: Pregnant woman in pink dress - laura-garcia (Pexels), Fetus model - Sinhyu (Adobe Stock Photos), IV saline - Anna-Shvets (Pexels), Group B streptococcus bacteria - cdc-sSVSWMa035g (Unsplash)

Week 36

There is very little room for the fetus inside the uterus. This makes it harder for the baby to give the mother kicks and punches.

However, you will still feel lots of stretching, rolling, and wiggling. If the baby hasn't already descended, it will now move into position for delivery.

Remember, just because it has descended does not mean you will start laboring. Give it time. From now on, you will most likely see your doctor every week until your baby is born.

What you can expect:

1. There is very little room for the fetus inside the uterus.
2. It is harder for the baby to kick.
3. You will still feel stretching, rolling, and wiggling.
4. If not already descended, it will now.
5. Remember, just because it has descended does not mean the labor will begin.
6. Give it time.
7. You will see the doctor every week until the birth.

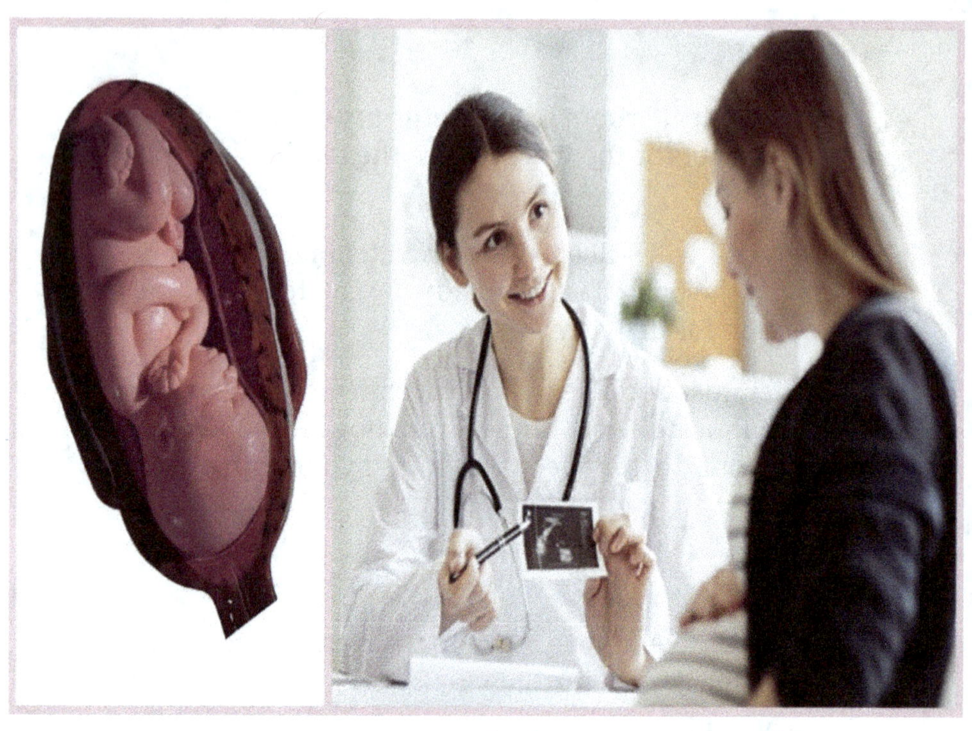

Image Credits: Fetus model - John Campbell (Wikimedia Commons - curid=99658179), Pregnant woman with Doctor - seventy four (Adobe Stock Photos)

Week 37

Your baby can grasp firmly now. The head or the buttocks (if the fetus is breech) might start descending into the pelvis.

Suppose your baby is not in a head-down position. In that case, your healthcare provider may recommend an "external cephalic version" procedure, where she will place her hands on your belly and, by pushing, try to turn your baby around into a head-down position.

Please do your research about this procedure and make your decision. Midwives are also trained to do this procedure as well. Some experienced midwives can also deliver a breech baby.

In a hospital, if the baby reverts to a breech position, the Obstetrician might recommend a C-section. It would be a good idea to brush up on your memory from your prenatal class videos and notes about Cesarean sections.

It is time to pack your baby bag with everything necessary to dress and bring the baby back home. Please pack the items you'd like to have to help manage the pain of labor and delivery.

What you can expect:

1. Baby can grasp firmly.
2. The head might start descending into the pelvis or the buttocks (if the fetus is breech.)
3. The doctor may recommend an "external cephalic version" procedure if not in a head-down position.
4. The doctor/Midwife places hands on your belly, pushes, and tries to turn your baby around.
5. Research this procedure and decide.
6. Experienced midwives can also deliver a breech.
7. In the hospital, if in a breech position, the Obstetrician might recommend a C-section.
8. Brush up on your notes about the Cesarean section.

9.   Keep the baby bag packed.

10. Pack up things you will need during the labor.

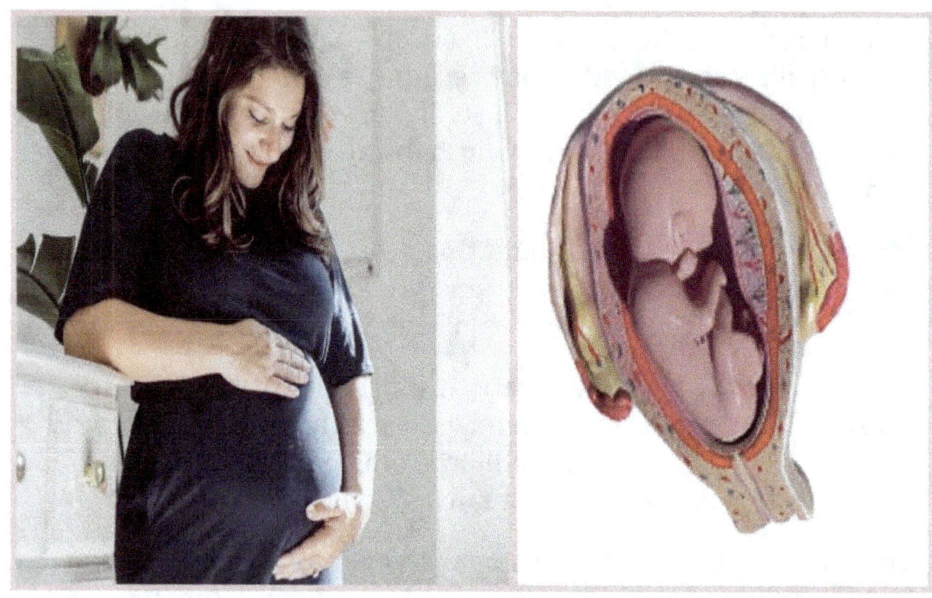

Image Credits: Pregnant Woman - amina-filkins-5427243 (Pexels), Fetus model - John Campbell (Wikimedia Commons - curid=99658182)

Week 38

There isn't much change in the baby's head and abdomen size. The toenails have grown full size, and the baby would have lost most of the lanugo hair.

"Early term" delivery is 37 weeks and 6 days into week 38.

Do your diligent research about stripping of membranes to start the labor early. It should be done only when it is necessary. Most of the time, it is not. And the procedure could be painful.

Though the chance of the baby being born perfectly healthy is higher during this week, most healthcare providers agree that it is best to let labor happen spontaneously.

From your prenatal class or through your doctor, you may have learned about what to do when you notice a "bloody show," if you begin having contractions that are strong and regular, or if your water bag breaks.

What you can expect:

1. No change in size.
2. Toenails - full size.
3. Lanugo - mostly gone.
4. "Early term" delivery = 37 weeks and 6 days into week 38.
5. Research about "stripping of membranes" to start labor early.
6. Should be done only when absolutely necessary.
7. The procedure could be painful.
8. Most of the time, it is not necessary.
9. Best to let labor happen spontaneously.
10. Learn about signs of labor: "bloody show," strong and regular contractions, and water bag breaks.

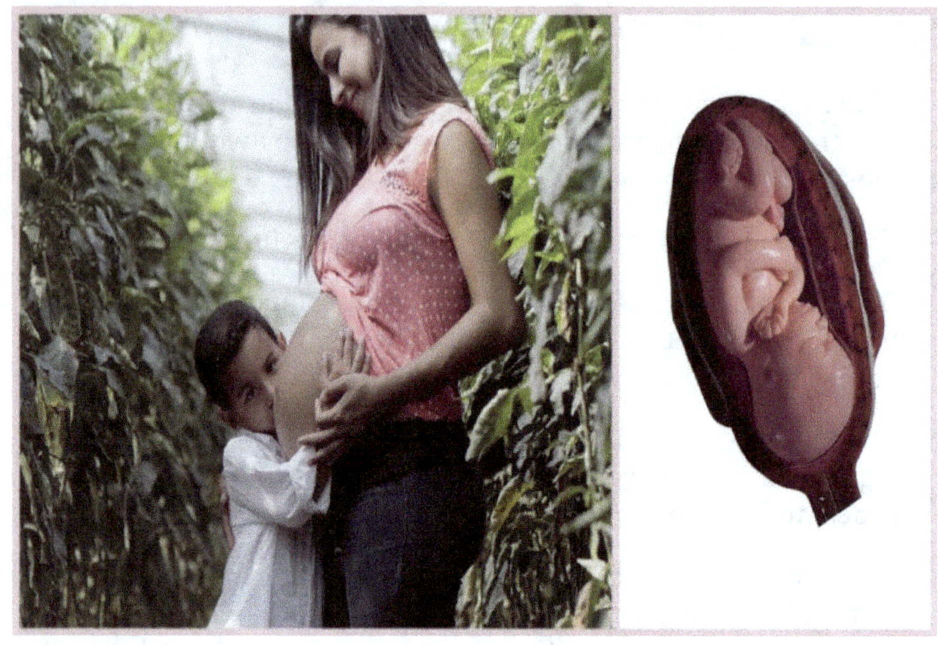

Image Credits: Boy kissing his mom's pregnant belly - Richard James (Unsplash), Fetus model - John Campbell (Wikimedia Commons - curid=99658179)

Week 39

Your baby's chest is developing more. If it is a boy, the testes would be descending into the scrotum. Fat is added all over the body to keep him or her warm after birth.

If your doctor suggests stripping of membranes, do your research first as to whether it is absolutely necessary. Most of the time, it's not. And the procedure could be painful.

If your baby were born during this week, he or she would have more than a 99 percent chance of being born perfectly healthy. However, unless there is a medical reason, it is better to wait for the labor to start spontaneously. Your baby might be needing just that little extra bit of time to develop more fully.

If you are scheduled to have a planned Cesarean, this might be the week your obstetrician may want to deliver your baby. Watch your prenatal class videos or read up on the subject to prepare yourself for the surgery.

What you can expect:
1. Your baby's chest is developing more.
2. Boy - the testes descend into the scrotum.
3. Fat to keep warm after birth.
4. If your doctor suggests stripping of membranes, do your research first as to whether it is absolutely necessary.
5. Most of the time, it is not, and the procedure could be painful.
6. Born during this week, 99 percent healthy.
7. However, it is better to wait for labor to start unless it is for medical reasons.
8. The baby might need a little extra time to develop fully.
9. If planned Cesarean: The obstetrician may want to deliver your baby this week.

10. Watch prenatal class videos or read about preparing for a C-section.

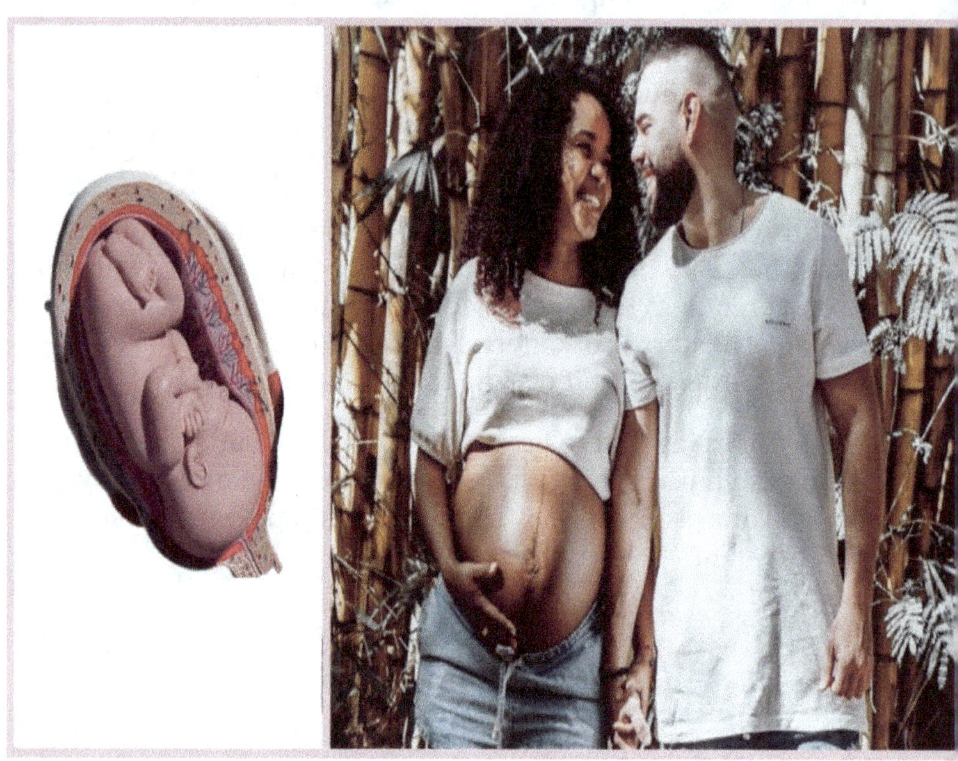

Image Credits: Fetus model - John Campbell (Wikimedia Commons - curid=99658182), Pregnant Couple - saulo-leite (Pexels)

Week 40

You have reached your due date! Your pregnancy is now considered full term - 39 weeks into the 40th week; your baby has an approximate length of around 14 inches -20 inches.

While weight might vary for each baby, as healthy babies come in different sizes, the baby will weigh approximately 6 to 8 pounds.

You could be meeting your baby any time now. Brush up on what you learned in your prenatal class about stages of labor and delivery, pain management, interventions, and unplanned C-sections. Go through your birth plan again. You got this!

What you can expect:

1. You have reached your due date!
2. Full term - 39 weeks into the 40th week.
3. Length is around 14 to 20 inches.
4. Weight might vary from 6 to 8 pounds.
5. Any time now!
6. Brush up points from prenatal class about stages of labor and delivery, pain management, interventions, and unplanned C-sections.
7. Go through the birth plan again.
8. You got this!

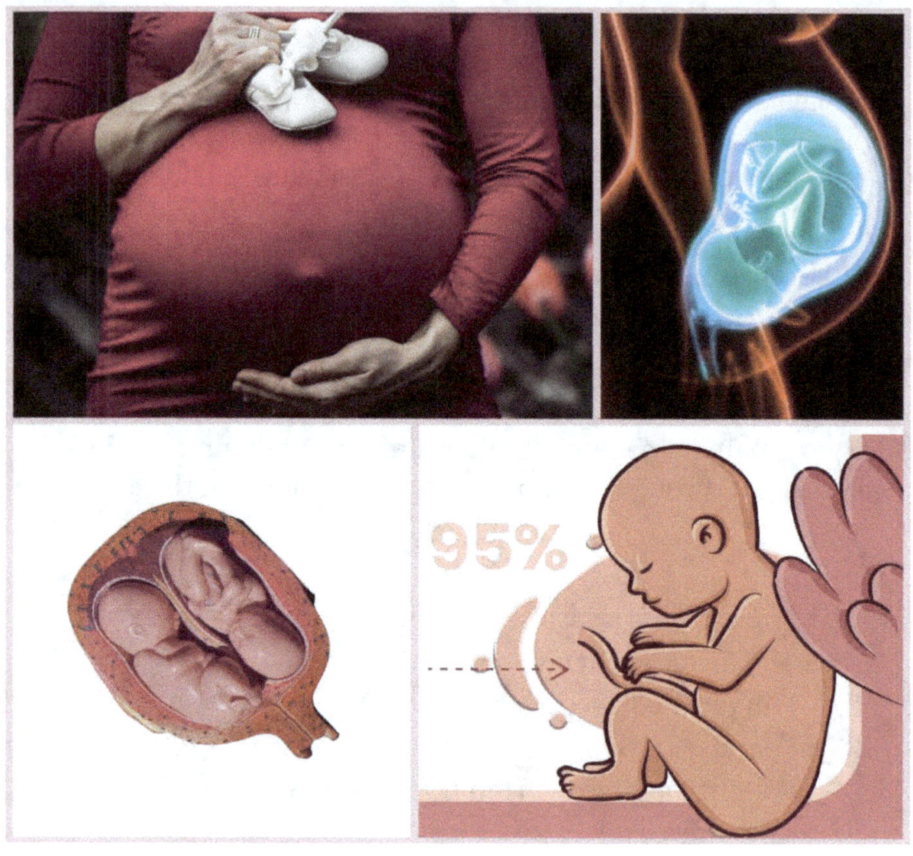

Image Credits: Pregnant belly at due date - Andre Furtado (Pexels), Fetus in a mother's belly - Magicmine (Adobe Stock Photos), Fetal Twins Model - John Campbell (Wikimedia Commons - curid=16229479398), 95% Fetus - Freepik

Week 41

Week 41 is called late-term. Don't forget that due dates are just those estimates and are never exact. The last thing you need is to worry unnecessarily. I suggest you go back to the due date from your first ultrasound, and your baby might most likely be on that schedule. My daughter went way past that due date.

If you are overdue, your doctor may want to see you twice a week for ultrasounds and fetal monitoring to ensure you and your baby are doing well.

Plan on getting as much rest as possible because soon, the marathon of labor, delivery, and taking care of the newborn will start. Conserve your energy and try to be as relaxed as possible. Keep practicing the labor positions, breathing, and relaxation techniques.

And talk to your baby. When you are calm, your baby will be calm. Keep sending "oxytocin" moments to the baby by sending love to your baby and expressing how excited you are to be meeting her/him soon.

What you can expect:

1. Week 41 = Late-term.
2. Don't forget that due dates are just estimates.
3. The last thing you need is to worry unnecessarily.
4. What was your due date from the first ultrasound?
5. Perhaps your baby is on that schedule.
6. If you are overdue, your doctor may want to see you twice a week for ultrasounds and fetal monitoring to check if you and the baby are doing well.
7. Get as much rest as you can. You are going to get very busy.
8. Conserve your energy, practice labor positions, breathing, and relaxation.

9. Talk to your baby - "Oh, I can't wait to see you soon, my baby!"

10. The baby can feel your emotions, so send "oxytocin" moments to the baby by sending love.

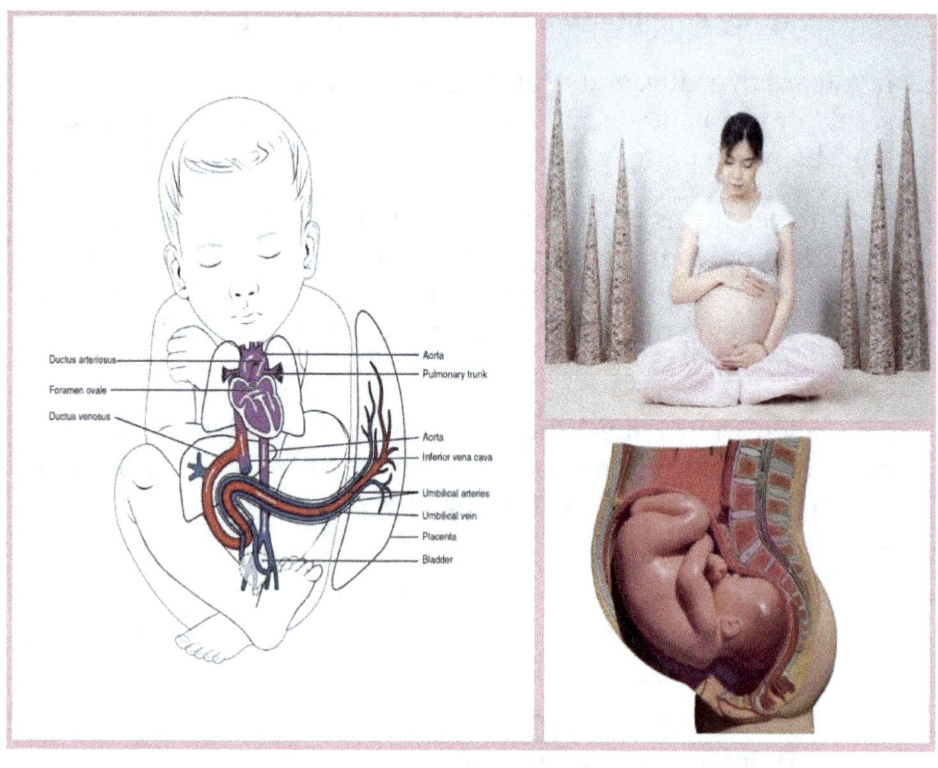

Image Credits: Circulatory System by OpenStax College - Anatomy & Physiology, Connexions (Wikimedia Commons - curid=30148296), Pregnant woman with a late-term belly - mikotoraw-photographer (Pexels), Fetus Model - John Campbell (Wikimedia Commons)

Week 42

Week 42 is called post-term. Though some midwives and birthing centers may allow the pregnancy to go beyond 42 weeks, your doctor may suggest induction at 42 weeks or even before that. It's a decision only you can make.

In the Netherlands, low-risk pregnancies are not allowed to be induced until they reach 42 weeks. But in the western world, especially in hospitals, it is not common practice to let the pregnancy go until 42 weeks. Do your research and make your decision. Remember, the calmer you are, the better decision you will make.

If you deliver in a hospital, the pediatrician may give your baby the first exam during the hospital stay. If you deliver in a birth center or at home, your pediatrician will want to see you within 48 hours of your baby's birth.

What you can expect:

1. Week 42 = Post-term.
2. Some midwives and birthing centers may allow the pregnancy beyond 42 weeks.
3. Your doctor may suggest induction at 42 weeks or even before that.
4. Remember, it's your decision.
5. In the Netherlands, low-risk pregnancies are not induced until 42 weeks.
6. In the West? Letting the pregnancy go until 42 weeks is not a common practice.
7. Do your research and make your decision.
8. Remember, the calmer you are, the better decision you will make.
9. The pediatrician may give the baby the first exam during the hospital stay.

10. At the birthing center or home, the pediatrician will see the baby within 48 hours of birth.

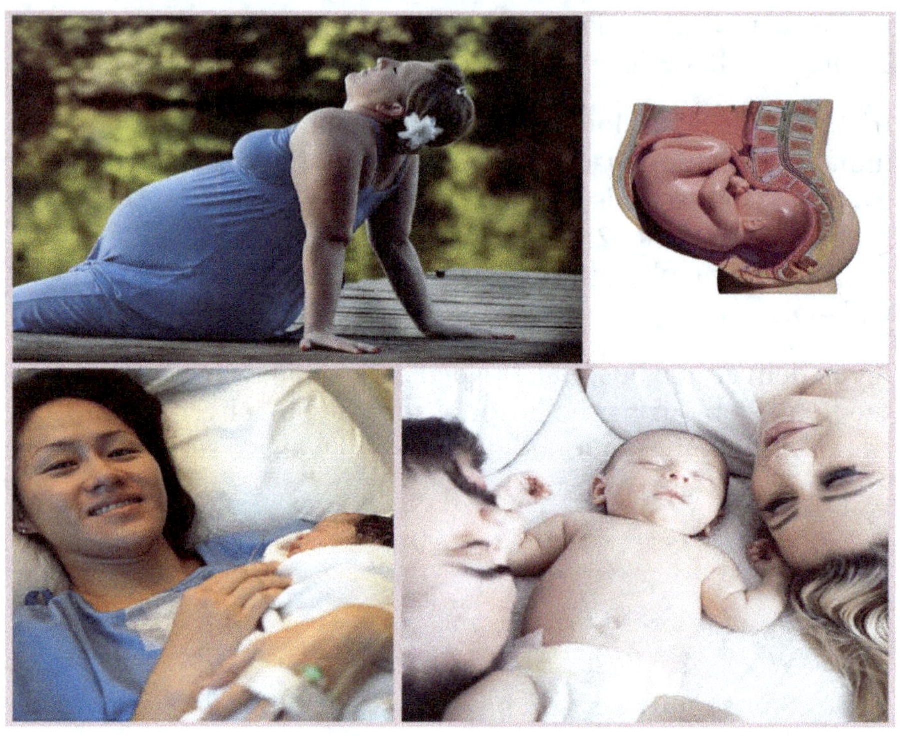

Image Credits: Post-term pregnant woman - Greyerbaby (Pixabay), Fetal Model - John Campbell (Wikimedia Commons), Mom with newborn child- blankita_ua (Pixabay), Couple with the baby - smpratt90 (Pixabay)

* * *

Dear Moms and dads, I know a new baby is a lot to take
on at once, but it's a great time to deepen your bond
with your newborn. I wish you all the best for a safe
and happy journey into parenthood.

Q.M. Sami, Mother, founder of Humsa Prenatals,
Childbirth Educator

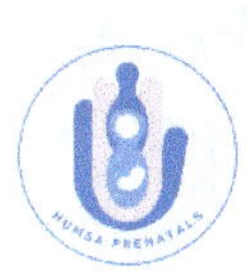

Learn More

To improve your pregnancy journey, all the chapters are now available in a video format on our https://www.youtube.com/@humsaprenatals

For an immersive experience, we bring you the All-in-one Labor, Delivery, Newborn Care, and Breastfeeding course on humsaprenatals.com.

If Webinars are your thing, we've got you covered with our affordable Master classes at humsaprenatals.com.

Week-by-Week Pregnancy Videos, Webinars, and More

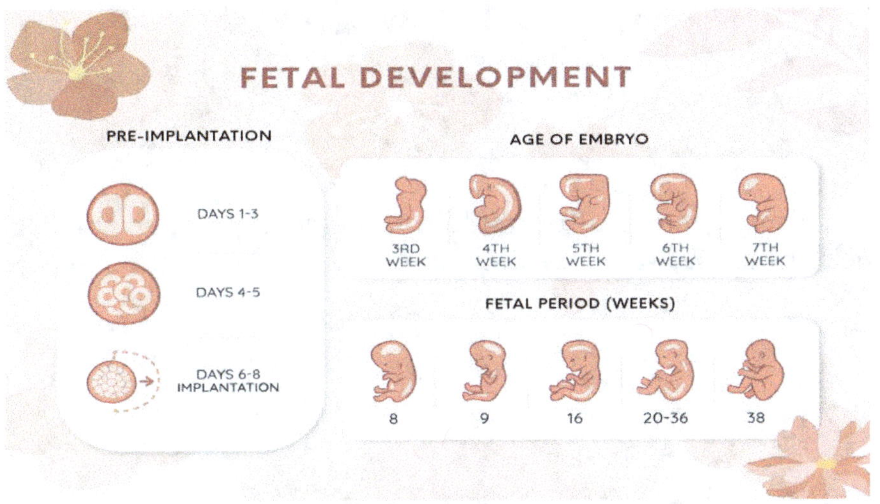

Humsa Prenatals aims to bring you the best pregnancy content. Explore all the chapters in their video format below.

FIRST TRIMESTER
YOUTUBE PLAYLIST

The first trimester starts on the first day of your last period and lasts until the end of week 12.

https://www.youtube.com/@humsaprenatals

SECOND TRIMESTER

YOUTUBE PLAYLIST

The second trimester is the middle part of your pregnancy, from weeks 13 to 27. https://www.youtube.com/@humsaprenatals

THIRD TRIMESTER

YOUTUBE PLAYLIST

The third trimester is the last phase of your pregnancy. It begins around week 28 and lasts until you give birth, that is till week 40, but sometimes it goes up to week 42.

https://www.youtube.com/@humsaprenatals

1. 10 chapters divided into 38 video sessions, each ranging from 3-15 minutes.
2. 19 real-life example videos that follow women through their birth experiences and their first steps into caring for their newborns.
3. You will learn about natural birth, epidural, C-section, self-care, care of the newborn, how to breastfeed, and much, much more.
4. The course is divided into an easy-to-remember format using simple questions: where, who, why, what, when, what if, what next, and how.

Make the best of your pregnancy! Enroll in the course now. A course that is totally geared to help you at every step of your journey through the process of labor, birth, and after.

Hear What Moms Have To Say:

"With all the free materials out there on YouTube, I was still struggling with finding the right content that would help me with my pregnancy journey. Right from the start, this course has kept me engaged and I got to learn so much from Miss Sami. Each lecture dwells deep into having a healthy pregnancy, the stages of labor and what to expect during that time, coping with pain, insights about epidural and pain medications, and taking care of ourselves. Not only that, Miss Sami even talks about dealing with postpartum depression and this is very important for a mother's mental health! This course gave me even more information about newborn care, from the hospital procedures to newborn screenings to help with baby sleep, baby's immunization, and even feeding techniques. I couldn't have asked for a better course on pregnancy, labor, and newborn care. Miss Sami is an extraordinary lecturer! Her soothing and calm tone made me want to spend more time listening to her lectures. I will highly recommend this course to all the new moms out there. If it's your first time and you want to know what to expect while expecting, look no further, Q.M. Sami's course is your pregnancy bible. This will truly be a great help for moms-to-be!"

Sameen Munir, Qatar

"This course provides information from the very beginning to the very end, and beyond. What to expect from the moment you get pregnant to the labour and beyond. It is very clear and to the point and provides different options available at different stages of the pregnancy. There are so many courses out there, and my partner and I are so happy and grateful, as this one includes all in one – all we needed to know – what to expect and what decisions to make, as we are first time parents. Thank you so much for all the valuable information. Your work is serving many of us!"

Dijana and Doruk, Toronto, Canada

"This course came as a recommendation from a friend. I can happily say that it has helped me with my pregnancy journey. Miss Sami is a great instructor, whose calming voice and paced speed, make this course even more soothing. I would recommend this course to women who are pregnant or who are planning to have a baby. Lots of information about pregnancy, newborn care, and more, packed in this one course. Hoping to see more content posted by Miss Sami. All the very best, ma'am!"

Sowmiya Prasad, Chennai, India

"Having a course that talks about all the aspects of labor, delivery, and newborn care has been really helpful. What's even better is the course being online and I can go through it at my own pace. Q.M. Sami has done a brilliant job with this course. I recommend this for new mothers or those who are planning to get pregnant and are in need of a simple and practical prenatal class."

R. Krishnan, Qatar

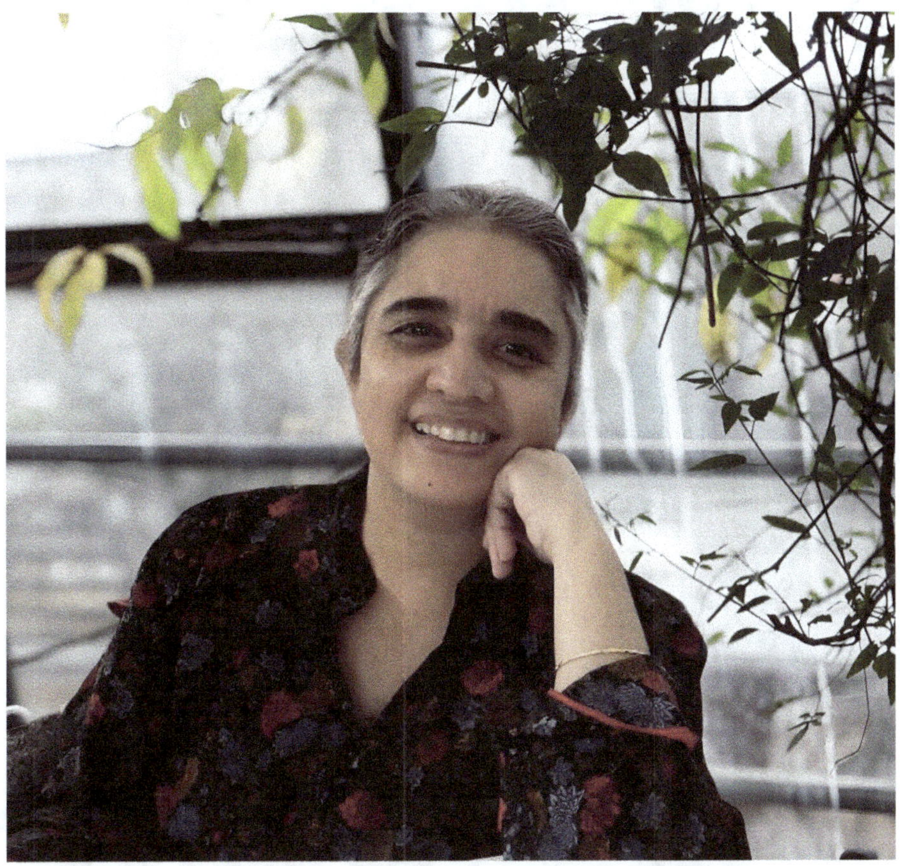

Q.M. Sami (B.Ed., PNSW, and DSW) is a Childbirth Educator, Content Creator, and the founder of Humsa Prenatals. Having worked with laboring mothers, Obstetricians, and Prenatal Educators, she gained a deep understanding of the struggles of pregnant women, especially in understanding and retaining the information and overcoming fears. She combined her experience as a mother and a Perinatal and Adult Educator to build and launch an online, self-paced, all-in-one Labor, Delivery, Newborn Care, and Breastfeeding course.

Check out the All-in-one Labor, Delivery, Newborn Care, and Breastfeeding course at https://humsaprenatals.com

You can also access the affordable Prenatal Webinars here.

Don't forget to check out the Week-By-Week Pregnancy Videos on https://www.youtube.com/@humsaprenatals

Social Media:

https://twitter.com/humsaprenatals

https://www.facebook.com/HumsaPrenatals

https://www.instagram.com/humsaprenatals

https://www.linkedin.com/company/humsa-prenatals

https://www.youtube.com/@humsaprenatals

www.ingramcontent.com/pod-product-compliance
Lightning Source LLC
Chambersburg PA
CBHW070837260726
48660CB00005B/2065